Angela Hobbs has written a poignant and highly personal account of her efforts to discover the causes of illnesses that she, and to a lesser degree her family, suffered from because of their home environment. Electrosensitivity, to the degree Mrs. Hobbs exhibited it, is fortunately not common, but her accounts of the multitudes of potentially hazardous exposures we all encounter in our homes is accurate and well presented. The most impressive part of her story is how in the face of physicians and even family telling her to see a psychiatrist she persisted and systematically tested factors in her home environment until she found the things that made her ill. This book is a pleasure to read, and will provide hope and a guide for action for those persons who suffer from unusual sensitivities to various environmental factors.

— DAVID CARPENTER, Director of the Institute for Health and the Environment, University at Albany and former Executive Secretary of the New York State Powerlines Project

Very impressive. *The Sick House Survival Guide* is very well organized and structured and the writing is vivid and engaging. Many electrically sensitive have become chemically sensitive and many chemically sensitive have become electrically sensitive — there is a complexity here — and the book deals with both phenomena in a very creative and helpful way. Highly recommended!

— LEIF SODERGREN, Swedish Association for the Electrically- and VDT-Injured (FEB)

The Sick House Survival Guide

The Sick House Survival Guide

Simple Steps to Healthier Homes

Angela Hobbs

NEW SOCIETY PUBLISHERS

Cataloguing in Publication Data
A catalog record for this publication is available from the National Library of Canada.

Cover design by Diane McIntosh. House image ©Eyewire.
Book and page layout design by Jeremy Drought, Last Impression Publishing Service.
Printed in Canada by Transcontinental Printing.

New Society Publishers acknowledges the support of the Government of Canada through the Book Publishing Industry Development Program (BPIDP) for our publishing activities.

Paperback ISBN: 0–86571–485–1

Inquiries regarding requests to reprint all or part of *The Sick House Survival Guide* should be addressed to New Society Publishers at the address below.

To order directly from the publishers, please add $4.50 shipping to the price of the first copy, and $1.00 for each additional copy (plus GST in Canada). Send check or money order to:

New Society Publishers
P.O. Box 189, Gabriola Island, British Columbia VOR 1X0, Canada
1 (800) 567•6772

New Society Publishers' mission is to publish books that contribute in fundamental ways to building an ecologically sustainable and just society, and to do so with the least possible impact on the environment, in a manner that models this vision. We are committed to doing this not just through education, but through action. We are acting on our commitment to the world's remaining ancient forests by phasing out our paper supply from ancient forests worldwide. This book is one step towards ending global deforestation and climate change. It is printed on acid-free paper that is 100% old growth forest-free (100% post-consumer recycled), processed chlorine free, and printed with vegetable based, low VOC inks.

For further information, or to browse our full list of books and purchase securely, visit our website at: www.newsociety.com

NEW SOCIETY PUBLISHERS
www.newsociety.com

Dedication

To Christopher and Richard

Table of Contents

Table of Illustrations

Photographs

Figures

Worksheets

Disclaimer

THIS GUIDE IS NOT INTENDED TO TAKE THE PLACE OF QUALIFIED MEDICAL ADVICE, but rather as a companion guide for creating a compatible healing environment. Any medical problems should be discussed with your family doctor — but choose your doctor carefully.

Acknowledgments

As I CRAWLED MY WAY BACK TO HEALTH, the people who cleared the rubble from my path took on significant importance. My parents, Judith and Sigvard von Sicard, gave me the gentlest of coaching. Bruce Small shared his philosophy of removing contaminant sources and Dr. William Ross Adey introduced me to the idea that chemicals and electromagnetic fields work together to undermine our health. Bonneville Power Administration sent me a free copy of the review by Dr. Jack Lee, Jr., "Electrical and Biological Effects of Transmission Lines" which revealed how many scientists have been working behind the scenes to make me well. My children, Christopher and Richard, glimmered as the light at the end of my tunnel.

When the idea of sharing my story and the eight steps to restore health became a possibility, several people made it a reality. My husband, Lawrence Hobbs, worked his magic on the computer. Errol Sharpe suggested my project to New Society Publishers where Christopher Plant saw its potential. Patricia Ludwick, my editor at New Society, polished the manuscript until it shone.

To all of you, my most sincere thanks.

Angela Hobbs
Calgary, Alberta
November 2002

Introduction

Hello and welcome to a new approach to creating a healthy home. You may have picked up this book out of sheer curiosity — how can houses be sick? Or you may experience strange symptoms yourself, and suspect they are connected to your home but not know what to do next. Like many of us, you may have received a diagnosis that does not make sense. You may well have been told your symptoms are psychosomatic — but if they were really caused by anxiety or depression, wouldn't you know what you were anxious or depressed about? Moving beyond a suspicion of our environment's role in our symptoms is a tremendous undertaking. The territory is largely uncharted: what little guidance is available suggests that we treat our sensitivities as allergies. Less than twenty years ago the United States Environmental Protection Agency (EPA) was asked to create a formal research program on indoor air quality. Today, officials at the National Institute for Occupational Safety and Health (NIOSH) recognize that we are still exposed to things in our homes that either have not yet been identified or that are not measured in a way that correlates them to health effects.[1] Such health effects include colds, influenza, allergies, asthma, sick building syndrome, etc.[2]

It's far easier to accept that our symptoms reflect internal disease than to prove that they are a reaction to the external environment. Doctors can treat our conditions if they are internal. However, if we suspect our symptoms may be a reaction to the environment, we are on our own: no one else will take responsibility for our health. Doctors have no solutions — which leaves the sick person alone to face isolation, despair, and sometimes even ridicule.

When we get sick we want to be able to rely on conventional medicine. We are taken in by its aura of complete success and have forgotten the role that preventative medicine, improved housing, sanitation, and immunization have played in that success.[3] The era when medical advances were made by considering the relationship between the environment and the creatures living in it — when we discovered the canary could warn coal miners of unsafe mines, or that milkmaids exposed to cowpox did not get smallpox — is long gone. Relationships like these led to the development of vaccines and measuring devices. Today's researchers overlook this kind of environmental connection. They see that sharks are cancer-free and that they avoid electromagnetic fields (EMFs), but instead of investigating the relationship between these two facts, they kill the shark and grind up its cartilage to use as medicine to fight cancer. What would we have done to the milkmaid had we discovered her in the 21st century?

There is still a great deal that conventional medicine can do. But guiding us through an analysis of our environment and the impact it has on our bodies is not one of its strengths. Doctors don't make house calls: they don't see us interacting with the environments in which we experience our symptoms. They simply cannot help us make connections.

This book will guide you through an analysis of your personal environment. It will show you how to pursue your symptoms and use your own tolerances to create an environment that is compatible for you. You will learn how to identify and reduce the many chemical and electromagnetic burdens on your body. With a few simple steps, you will be able to replace those feelings of defeat with feelings of strength. You will learn enough about the connection between electromagnetic fields, chemicals, hormones, and health to enable you to gain control over your symptoms. This approach to creating a compatible environment within your own home will cost you nothing and may very well save you money, time, and suffering.

Wouldn't it be lovely to discover that the depression you wake up with every morning — the one that leaves you sitting in a puddle of tears and doesn't lift until lunch — is related to the position of your bed in a pocket of electromagnetic fields? Wouldn't you love to discover that your heart palpitations at the store checkout, are your body's response to the concoction created by cleaning aisle odors and the power at the check out. Wouldn't you feel totally empowered if you discovered that if you took a few paces to the left, you might walk right out of the pocket of electromagnetic fields responsible for the panic attack that's about to take hold of you? If your symptoms are related to your environment, you may well be about to discover, as I did, that relief is as readily accessible as that.

This book is divided into three sections:

Part 1 tells my story — my triumph over the symptoms that led doctors to suspect some of medicine's cruelest diseases. Unable to recognize the connection between my symptoms and my highly toxic environment, the very professionals on whom I relied were powerless to help. To heal, I had to let my symptoms guide me. Eventually, I had to overcome the idea that there is a "safe" distance from the appliances in my home.

Part 2 will take you through eight Simple Steps — an approach to creating a healing environment. You will learn how electromagnetic fields affect your body's ability to deal with chemicals, how to recognize sources of chemicals and electromagnetic fields, and how and *when* to reduce them.

Part 3 looks at some of the measures other countries are taking to mitigate the dangers of electromagnetic fields. It also suggests some ways of reducing your exposure in your own neighborhood.

In the US alone, millions of people report chronic symptoms like headaches, fatigue, and joint or muscle pain — which have no obvious cause.[4] Clearly there is a need for a closer look at the environments in which such symptoms develop. Until now, treatment has focused either on reducing chemicals or on maintaining a safe distance from appliances. Ironically, several of the authors who recommend one or another of these approaches are themselves still struggling to overcome their symptoms. My hope is that by combining these approaches, you will return, as I did, to full and vibrant health.

Part One

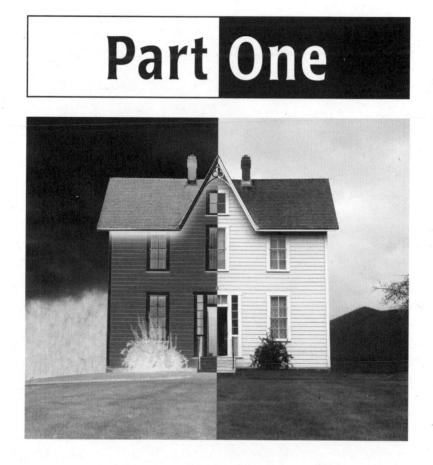

1

The Start of Something New

WHEN I MOVED TO ONTARIO IN THE SPRING OF 1996, I was a healthy thirty-five-year-old wife and the mother of two little boys. Christopher was six at the time and Richard was three. Our days were filled with active living; we all loved walking, swimming, and cycling. After the difficulties we had had having our children, I was thrilled that we were all so healthy. I could definitely give myself a pat on the back — I was doing a good job.

Developing Symptoms

As my husband, Lawrence Hobbs, and I watched the moving van drive away and shut the door on our new house in Newmarket, Ontario, we gave a huge sigh of relief. We had no idea that the experience that lay ahead would be a far cry from what we anticipated. We were blissfully unaware of the many dangers harbored by our new home.

The beautiful house that would soon begin to cause our problems was a fully renovated older home. The kitchen and bathrooms had new cabinetry and linoleum, a new pale gray carpet ran through the living room and up the stairs, opening onto newly varnished wood floors in four bedrooms. Every inch of the house had had a fresh lick of paint. Every room had that lovely new smell. We had chosen the house carefully: the renovations would eliminate the need for maintenance, the small garden wouldn't demand much care, and the high water table ensured a succulent lawn without much watering.

Disorientation

As the summer came to an end, the children went off to school and Lawrence to work, leaving me to unpack our boxes and settle into our new home. I breathed the new smell day and night, and by the end of the first week I began to feel quite disoriented. After two weeks the new smell began to seem more caustic than fresh, and by the end of the third week I had become forgetful. I would forget to do the most basic things, such as shopping for groceries, making beds, washing dishes, and getting supper, and I was unable to make any headway at all with the boxes I was supposed to be unpacking. By the end of the third month in our house, I even forgot to pick up the children from school.

At that point, nothing about my house resembled any of my former homes — the Martha Stewart in me was definitely out to lunch. I was living in a pigsty: the laundry hamper was overflowing, the kitchen was littered with dirty dishes, and the beds hadn't seen clean sheets in over a month. There wasn't a curtain in sight and not even a mouse could have found supper in my fridge.

Dizziness

With no curtains on our big picture windows, we felt something like the proverbial goldfish. I had planned to make curtains for all the windows once the boxes were unpacked, but after three months we couldn't wait any longer. We went out and bought full-length rubberized curtains for the living room and master bedroom and Lawrence helped me to unwrap them and hang them up. We felt the rubberized material would help with drafts and maybe cut down on the cost of heating with electric baseboards.

By the time the curtains were up, I was dizzy and by morning, I was positively heaving. Much to Lawrence's annoyance I was convinced that it was the curtains were making me dizzy — they had to come down. Somewhat annoyed at my suspicions, Lawrence helped take down the curtains but made me promise to see a doctor because he was adamant that "curtains don't make you sick."

Anxiety?

My first visit to a doctor left me with a diagnosis of anxiety. Blood tests revealed I was in perfect health and all the doctor could suggest was that I pamper myself and ride it out — the anxiety would soon pass.

Somewhat reassured, I went home and washed my new curtains, ironed them carefully, and hung them up. But by morning I was heaving and dizzy and down they came again. Clearly we would have continue our lives as goldfish and not use the curtains until my anxiety abated.

As I waited for my anxiety to pass I tried to control my disorientation and forgetfulness by dividing my day into chunks and focusing my attention on specific tasks. I drew up a checklist to refocus myself; each morning I would check off the activities I accomplished. In the morning, I tidied up, made the beds, and unpacked a box. After lunch I would take a walk and unpack another box, making sure to finish in time to pick up the children. But try as I might, I accomplished very little and still managed to forget to collect the boys from school at least a couple of times a week.

Caustic Odors

As the fourth month began, the smell in my house really started to bother me. I would notice it as soon as I walked into the house and it would linger at the back of my throat with pungency, like the smell of the skunks that my dog had chased in Quebec. The smell became increasingly less fresh and more caustic and no longer faded with time as it had in the early days.

I tried to locate where this caustic smell was coming from, sniffing my way from item to item. Everything seemed to have a smell but the worst offenders appeared to be the wood floors in the bedrooms. Washing them had little impact on the smell, so I started covering them with blankets. I hoped that by doing this I could absorb the smell and prevent it from getting into the air, especially at night. Initially the smell would be contained, but after a few hours the blankets would be saturated. I would gather them up and hang them outside to air. I'd replace them with other blankets, sheets, anything absorbent that wasn't being used on the beds. The procedure was arduous and I was soon on the phone to the manufacturers of the varnish to find out if there was anything else I could do. The manufacturers suspected that the wood floors had been refinished in a hurry and not left to cure between coats. They told me that each coat of urethane needed to dry out for several days before the next layer. They assured me that if I ventilated well, the smell would probably be gone within a year — but in the meantime the smell was toxic.

"Toxic" was a familiar word: I'd heard it in relation to toxic waste and mixing cleaning solutions, but now "toxic" was in all of our bedrooms. Worst of all, it was in the bedrooms of my innocent children who were relying on me to keep them safe. This was the first of my many challenges from the multiple dangers hidden in my house, and I ventilated with abandon. Every time I opened a window my disorientation decreased, and every time I closed them, it would increase. So, as much for myself as for my children, I wanted to find a quick way to get rid of the chemicals that were offgassing from the wood floors. Opening windows seemed like a very short-term solution.

I rented a huge industrial extractor fan and set it up in the basement. I attached a long cardboard tube so that it blew any indoor air right out of the basement window. With all the windows open throughout the house and all the doors propped open I turned the machine on. Within half an hour it had removed all the caustic-smelling air — and along with it, my disorientation. For a couple of hours I was functional in my house: I could unpack and remember where I'd put just about everything. But by evening, the smell was back and I was as dysfunctional as ever. Though the extractor fan made an impression, it was an expensive alternative to window ventilation.

Lawrence had heard about heating as a means of speeding the process of offgassing and several times we tried to "bake" the house in an effort to speed the offgassing process. We turned on all the electric baseboard units, shut all the windows, and left. The house baked for four hours before we came home and ventilated. After several sessions we realized that the impact we were having on the smell was negligible. While it is possible to increase the offgassing from one item by applying heat, when you're talking about removing the chemicals from a whole house, the amount of heat, expense, and time involved is simply daunting.

"Toxic" was still in our bedrooms and I needed more than open windows to get rid of it, so next I tried a dehumidifier. I knew that things don't smell as bad in dry air. So maybe if I could dry the air in the house the smell wouldn't bother me as much. I was stunned at the amount of water the dehumidifier sucked up — only to learn that there was an underground stream just inches below our basement floor. That explained both the dampness and why the sump pump was going all the time. Obviously, all the dehumidifier would accomplish was changing the course of the stream – up into the bucket and down the toilet.

The dehumidifier had little impact on the smell: if anything it added to the EMFs around me. The only thing left to try was air fresheners. Maybe if I could change the smell, my disorientation would go away. Little did I realize that by adding air fresheners, I was compounding the problem with yet more chemicals.

Head Swellings

During my battle with the toxic offgassing of my wood floors I developed jaw pains and began losing my balance. My battle with the wood floors was brought to an abrupt halt when the children caught back-to-school colds and had to stay home. Richard's cold became strep throat and Christopher's became bronchitis which left them home on antibiotics for three weeks.

This was the first time since their ear infections as babies that my children had been on antibiotics. The problem now, though, was that with two sick kids I could hardly be opening the windows to air out the house. What I needed to do was close the windows and turn up the heat to keep them nice and cozy. I fought hard to keep the "toxic" from the wood floors from entering our air, by covering them with blankets which I changed frequently, but I still found the smell terrible. With my lack of balance, disorientation, and jaw pains I was almost as sick as the children.

The antibiotics caused both Christopher and Richard to have severe diarrhea, and consequently the washer and dryer were on all the time. In this warm, cozy, unventilated house with the washer and dryer going full tilt, I was introduced to the first of what I came to call "head swellings." Standing in the kitchen dosing the children with their medicine, I began to feel my head swelling up. The excruciating pressure continued to build until I thought I'd scream, and then, just as suddenly as it had begun, I felt a pop and the eeriest sensation of water trickling down my spine.

Diagnoses

As soon as the children were back at school, I took myself off to the doctor again. I described the buildup of pressure in my head, the pop, and the subsequent trickle down my spine. I complained again about my disorientation and forgetfulness. I told her about my lack of balance and I described the pain and the constant clicking in my jaw that had all developed in the last two months. But the doctor couldn't see my profound level of disorientation — I didn't seem to be having any problems with it that she could see. Nor could she see the excruciating pressure and paralyzing fear that came with my head swellings. The doctor dismissed the clicking in my jaw as a dental issue, a specific disorder that lay outside the parameter of her expertise which was therefore eliminated from her consideration. From where the doctor stood, the symptoms — for which I had no evidence — had to be in my mind: an expression of anxiety. The doctor suggested I pamper myself and relax a little; she assured me that in time my symptoms would pass.

The Dentist

Since the doctor had been very clear that my jaw problems were a dental issue, I called my dentist and made an appointment. Maybe the dentist would be able to give me some exercises or suggestions to help alleviate some of the discomfort in my jaw. My dentist saw me quickly; I was, after all a lucrative patient who just months earlier had a full set of x-rays and four mercury amalgam fillings replaced because of cavities. Unfortunately, however, the dentist could do little to help me. She advised me that I had Temporal-Mandibular Joint Syndrome (TMJ) and would need an operation to file down the bone that was causing the clicking and clunking. She had no idea why it hadn't shown up in my earlier x-rays. Neither the doctor nor the dentist were willing to consider that my jaw problem and my disorientation might be connected. To me, they were both in my head, but to these accredited professionals, they were in different parts of my head and each signified a different condition.

The Blackout

I tried to follow the doctor's advice: to relax, pamper myself, and think about other things. But the symptoms didn't pass — they grew worse. Many of my meals were soft or eaten through a straw — when I didn't totally forget them. The head swellings came at least thirty times a day. I was often so disoriented that the school would have to call me to come and get my children; several times the children just didn't get to school. Lawrence would come home to supper only to be greeted by, "Oh, is it that time already?"

The beginning of the fifth month in our house brought Christopher's seventh birthday. I wanted it to be special and I really pushed myself into preparation mode. I invited our neighbors over for cake and coffee; their kids could help to whack the piñata. Once the invitations were out, I had to get things ready. I loaded the children into the car and set off for the local department store. Feeling rather stressed, I raced around the store picking up birthday essentials. I found the birthday candles and a couple of little goodies for their new friends. But I kept forgetting what I was doing at the store and became increasingly disoriented and confused. The expedition ended disastrously. I have a vague recollection of standing at the checkout with my checkbook trying to hold the sum on the cash register in my head long enough to write the total on the check. The next thing I remember is sitting in my car with my children and no packages. According to Christopher, he had lead me out of the store by my hand, like a child. I hugged my children tight and sobbed as I realized that I could quite easily have left them behind with the shopping.

I felt a surge of panic as I realized the danger I had put my children in. I had had to rely on my six-year-old child to take care of me! It wasn't right that he should have to lead me out of a store. It wasn't right that I could black out like this if nothing was wrong. If this indeed was anxiety then I had to take it very seriously. Until it abated, it wouldn't be safe for me to go out with my children alone.

So this birthday would have no piñata, but I did manage a cake — a chocolate castle populated by Lego knights, both good guys and bad. There would be plenty of juice and coffee and there would be another call to the doctor and another appointment. Surely now the doctor would help me. I'd had the perfect opportunity to focus on something other than myself but whatever was wrong with me affected every aspect of my life. Every day that passed I was less functional — and now I'd even had a blackout.

Seizures

By the time I returned to the doctor I had developed several other symptoms. I'd begun shaking at night, my right arm was constantly tingling and would often shrivel up and turn purple, and I'd start to cry or laugh on the outside even though I didn't feel that way inside. I described my new symptoms to the doctor, especially the shaking that would start with my body going into a spasm followed by a gentle vibration, similar to the vibration of a tumble dryer. At the time I didn't recognize this as a seizure but the doctor seemed more concerned than previously. She gave me another physical and when she thought she could feel a lump in my womb, she sent me for an internal ultrasound. She asked me to get Lawrence to watch my shaking and record it for her. If someone else could see the symptoms, then maybe they weren't all in my head.

To ask Lawrence to stay up to watch my shaking after a day's work, a three-hour commute, and a sink full of dishes, was like making a sleeping child walk. By the time he went to bed he had also had to deal with dirty laundry, making the beds, filling the fridge, ironing his shirts, and generally trying to make some sense of the total disarray he came home to. We tried several times, though: I would lie in my bed and try to go to sleep while he stood over me, lights blaring, waiting for me to start shaking. We laughed plenty; the situation was comical, if only it hadn't been so terribly frightening. As soon as the lights were out and the weight of sleep descended on me, the tightening and trembling would begin, but by then Lawrence was already asleep.

Disbelief

"Perfect Health"

I'd been in my house for five and a half months when I went back to the doctor for the results of my ultrasound. By now my days began with vomiting and I sweated profusely during the night, so much so that I would have to change my bed at least twice a night. I was a real mess and I hoped that either the ultrasound or the blood tests would reveal something that could be treated. I was convinced that I had a tumor in my womb and I was ready for the doctor to tell me the worst. But again, to my relief, disappointment, and utter confusion, I was "fine." The ultrasound had revealed nothing: there was no lump in my womb. Blood tests showed that

I was in perfect health and since I didn't have any confirmation of my seizures, the doctor could only assume that they were a figment of my imagination. She concluded again that I must be suffering from a very bad case of anxiety.

"Anxiety" — Oh, Really?

It was difficult for Lawrence to understand what was going on. He wasn't home much because his job and commute kept him in downtown Toronto until late in the evening. Spending barely any time in the house, he was unaffected by the odors and pretty much thought that I was being rather silly and obsessive. He must have been able to see how sick I was; certainly I complained plenty. But since the doctor had said that my only problem was anxiety which she was confident would pass, I guess he was just ready to wait it out. In his eyes he had excelled as a provider: he had set us up in a great community and in a beautiful house. Now he had to keep us there by commuting to downtown Toronto. He just felt frustrated that I wasn't getting the house sorted out. He was used to coming home to a hot meal, a tidy house, happy children, and ironed shirts. He found himself coming home instead, to a crying wife, an unmade bed, dirty washing, an empty fridge, no supper, and his children glued to the television.

But could this really be anxiety? It seemed to me that I'd been in plenty of situations where anxiety would have been warranted — losing Christopher at Chicago airport, nursing two children through chicken pox in a hotel, losing my dog in transit between Montreal and Kansas — why hadn't I felt this anxiety then? What about when the bush pilot bringing us down from arctic Quebec in his Twin Otter had had to jump his plane off the cliff because the runway was too short? I'd been in plenty of situations where a reaction of anxiety would have been understandable, but there was nothing about my new situation that warranted this kind of debilitating anxiety. I had a couple of years ahead of me in which to straighten out my certification that would allow me to teach in Ontario; I had new friends and a beautiful home. There was just nothing about my new situation that I was anxious about. So I decided that maybe I needed to see another doctor. If nothing else, I would then have a second opinion.

Psychiatrist or Tranquilizers?

I described my symptoms to the new doctor: how the extractor fan had alleviated my disorientation, how I reacted to the fumes in my house, and how I felt my symptoms were far more manageable when I was out. I asked him if there was any possibility that my symptoms could be related to the fumes from the wood floors. After more blood tests the new doctor simply decided I was suffering from "stress." He could offer me tranquilizers, but he thought I would do better to see a psychiatrist. I could count on one hand the pills that I had taken in the whole of my life and tranquilizers were simply not an option. So I went home and told Lawrence that the new doctor recommended I see a psychiatrist.

At this stage I spent many days shrunk into a corner sobbing and holding my head, just begging the head swellings to stop. Maybe the doctors were right: maybe this was all in my mind. Maybe, if nothing else, I had become anxious about being anxious. I was frightened at the repercussions that seeing a psychiatrist could have. I envisioned myself being heavily drugged at best and at worst committed to an institution. In a desperate effort I tried to talk to Joan, an old friend who had known me before this all started. She'd helped me with my children over the years and she was smart, scared of doctors, and a trusted friend. I lead Joan through my house, getting her to sniff the air in the basement, the ground floor, and the bedrooms. I hoped that she would react to something, but to no avail. Instead, Joan assured me that there was nothing wrong with my house and that I should follow the advice of the doctor and make an appointment with the psychiatrist.

The Snowball Effect

So there were four people — two doctors, my husband, and my friend — who were all thinking clearly and all telling me to see a psychiatrist. There was no way that smells could be making me as sick as I was and the incident with the curtains was simply coincidence. Every time that I complained about my symptoms, Lawrence and Joan would become more adamant that I needed to see a psychiatrist and would push harder for me to make an appointment. Each time their arguments would seem more rational and I would feel less convinced that my gut feeling about the fumes had any foundation. They could see I was sick, and thought that following the course of conventional medicine was the only way to get me help. As I left Lawrence and Joan to talk into the night, I was overcome by visions of *One Flew Over the Cuckoo's Nest*. What would happen to my children? Who would take care of my beautiful little boys? I loved them so much and now they would never know the real me — how devoted I'd been to them and how their lives had defined my very existence. They would see me only as "that crazy woman." They'd go through their lives wondering if I'd passed it on!

Is Anxiety Hereditary?

I spent days trying to weigh both sides of the argument. Could it be that these symptoms were an expression of anxiety? Had they been passed on by my mother and father? Much as I didn't want them worrying about me, I needed to talk to them. I needed to know if this anxiety was hereditary and if anyone else in the family had suffered from it. Before I let the snowball gather too much speed, I had to talk to my parents. Mum and Dad had always worked together as one. As missionaries who had raised three children in the African bush, they had certainly experienced anxiety. They were the only people that I could really trust to help me. I knew that they always held my best interests close to their hearts. I picked up the phone and I called Mum.

Of course Mum and Dad were concerned and they were ready to jump into the car there and then. There was no question in the minds of these seventy-year-old people about undertaking the twelve-hour drive from their summer home in Maine. I felt so desperate that my whole body was screaming, "Yes, please come!" and I so wanted to say it aloud. But if they saw me like this they would be devastated; it would break their hearts. I simply had to have some time to get ready for them — I had to get better before they came.

Of all the things we chatted about Mum made one thing absolutely clear: she had never experienced symptoms like mine. Any time Mum had experienced stress or anxiety, she had always known what it was about. "You don't just get anxious, Angela," she said, "You get anxious about something."

In the days that followed, these words repeated themselves over and over again in my head. It was a relief to know my symptoms weren't hereditary and that they weren't typical of anxiety. But most of all, it was a relief to know that Mum and Dad would soon be coming up to see me. I could hold out until they came. Maybe I could stop the snowball from gathering any more momentum if

I stopped talking about my symptoms. I could tell Lawrence and Joan that I was going to let my parents see me before I committed myself to anyone's care. I could hold on to Mum's words as they echoed in my head and gave me strength. "You don't just get anxious, Angela. You get anxious about something."

During the two weeks that followed I worked hard to get my home and myself ready for Mum and Dad's visit. If I couldn't get the boxes unpacked, at least I could stack them neatly. If I couldn't get the laundry done, at least it could be in the hampers. But as I worked I noticed a severe weakening in my right arm. No longer was it just shriveling: it was so weak that I couldn't change the gears in my standard car.

The Trip

Lawrence quickly noticed that I had stopped talking about my symptoms — that I hadn't really said anything about anything since his last push for me to make an appointment with the psychiatrist. Unwilling to spend the weekend with my silence, Lawrence made arrangements to visit our old friends, Betty and Rick, who'd recently moved from Montreal to Cambridge, Ontario. This was the first time that we had left Newmarket since the beginning of the school term and I really wasn't sure that I was up to it. If I didn't agree to go, the debate about my symptoms would be reopened — I would be pushed closer to the edge and closer to the psychiatrist. I had resolved to hold out until my parents came and I had more to lose by not going than by going.

What was utterly amazing about this little trip was its effect on me. I suddenly felt fine. It was drastic. One minute my head was swelling and I was alternately crying and laughing hysterically, and the next I was my old self. I could hold a conversation with Lawrence for the first time in two months. I could follow a thought through from start to finish, I could laugh at the appropriate time, and I didn't suddenly burst into tears for no apparent reason. I could hardly believe it, but I felt fine. We had a wonderful day, one that left me totally confused. Could it be that my stress had left me? Could it be that in these five months of hell all I needed to do was to see an old friend? Could it be that I really wasn't going to end up in a psychiatric hospital? It was probably too early to tell, but one thing I knew for sure: I felt great.

I spent a lot of time in Betty's bathroom furiously writing myself notes. It was here that I realized just how disoriented I had become. I realized there was a good chance that my symptoms were a response to something in my environment rather than an illness: after all, my environment was the only thing I had changed in coming out to Cambridge. A seed of hope was planted deeper in my mind than any symptoms could reach. As the seed germinated I felt that, though I might be looking for a needle in a haystack, there was a chance that my body wasn't getting sick all by itself, but rather in response to something in my environment.

I decided that if the symptoms returned when I got home, I would go on seeing doctors until I could get some specific help and a specific diagnosis. There might be some who would laugh and there would be others who would push anxiety at me. Maybe some of my problem stemmed from anxiety, but there was something else going on, too. There had to be somebody out there who would be able to help me. I was going to have to hunt, but I was going to find some answers.

Home Again

As we approached our housing development in Newmarket, all my symptoms came flooding back full force. For several days I was so sick I couldn't even get out of bed. Christopher didn't go to school because I couldn't get him there. He took care of Richard; how he found anything for them to eat I'll never know. I depended totally on this little seven-year-old child.

What else was I to do? I didn't know anyone well enough to ask for help. My new friends weren't in any position to help me since Laura was getting over a miscarriage and Lynn was having chest pains that were soon to be diagnosed as late-onset asthma. Lawrence and Joan seemed ever anxious to have me committed; I felt that asking them for help would only hasten my removal to an institution. I needed time so badly; I just longed to go back to Betty's house so my head would be clear enough to work this out. I needed someone to believe that this wasn't all in my mind and that there was more to it than simply treating the symptoms. Again I held on to Mum's words, "You don't just get anxious, Angela. You get anxious about something." I held on to the knowledge that Mum and Dad were coming. And I held on to the hands of Christopher and Richard. If I could just keep my mouth shut about my symptoms for a few more days, however bad it got, then Mum and Dad would help me. They had to!

The little hand that reached for me now was the same little hand that had rocked my shoulder when the pain of a sick premature baby had been too much to bear. Just as he had come to claim me when Richard was in the hospital, Chris came to claim me now. Deep in his beautiful eyes I could see fear, in his hand I could feel that he would not let go. I was Mummy, he needed breakfast, and if I could just set him up with a nice show, he would take care of Richard.

Hope

It was the end of my sixth month in Newmarket when my parents arrived. I had managed to pull myself out of bed on Saturday morning and their beds were ready. There was no way that they would recognize my house as the house of their very organized daughter, but there was nothing I could do about it. When I opened the door to welcome them after their twelve-hour drive, I couldn't hold back the tears of relief and hope. I fell into their arms pleading, "You have to help me Mum, Dad, you have to help me, nobody believes me."

Despite the late hour, my parents sat me down in the living room. They could see by the disorganization around them and my weight loss that something was really wrong. The vivacious, energetic daughter who had spent a week with them early in the summer, swimming, jogging, and playing with the children, was not the person sitting on the sofa. I listened as Lawrence filled them in on the doctors' reports. As he saw the problem, I was refusing the treatment that they had recommended and I was getting sicker by the day. He'd tried to help me get rid of the smell that I was always complaining about but felt powerless to help. I had put so much hope into my parents being able to help me, but as I listened to Lawrence's very rational explanation, I suddenly felt overwhelmed. What if they agreed? What if they were unwilling to explore the possibility that my body was reacting to something in my environment? Of everyone in the world, Mum and Dad were the ones that I would listen to. They had stood by me through so much. If they told me to see a psychiatrist, then I would.

But they didn't. They sat in my living room very quietly watching my every breath. When they had heard the whole story from Lawrence, they turned to me. They asked me what I felt was wrong. I told them that I felt there was something really wrong with my house. I told them about feeling great in Cambridge and I told them I felt there was a terrible smell that I couldn't get rid of, and that the smell made me wish, with all my heart, that I could just run away and never come back.

My parents sent us out for a walk. They needed time to go over what we'd said, to adjust to the shock that they might only just have arrived in time. They needed to work out their plan. As I got up to go, I hugged my Dad; he held with the same strength that had comforted me as a child. "Please help me, Dad, nobody believes me."

"Run, Angie, Run"

When we returned, Mum and Dad had taken over. They greeted us at the door and handed me my toothbrush, pajamas, and a change of clothes. They were giving me the chance to run away — temporarily, but for long enough to find out if my gut feeling was right. I was to go and stay at a motel until I could think clearly and cope with my situation. I didn't need to be told twice. I didn't even show them their beds. These two wonderful people in their seventies were going to take over my house and take care of my children, at eleven o'clock at night after a twelve-hour drive. Of course, they might still decide that a psychiatrist was the only option, but they would give me every chance to get better first.

So I left my house, bag in hand. I would not return for three days and I prayed with all my heart that God would give me the strength to get to the bottom of my troubles and show me the path to the source of this "anxiety."

2

Coping with the Symptoms

Finding My Way

AS WE REACHED THE MOTEL AT AROUND MIDNIGHT, Lawrence seemed to forget the reason behind the trip. He went into honeymooner mode — no kids, motel, wife to himself — and yet only two hours earlier, he'd been graphically explaining my condition to my parents and had taken me out for a walk that I could barely complete. Somewhat annoyed with what he'd come to see as my obsession, he went to bed. I, on the other hand, sat up late into the night. For a whole week I'd been so sick I hadn't been able to get out of bed. In the motel my head was clear; I didn't have a single head swelling and I fell asleep without fever or shaking.

When I awoke, Lawrence had already left for work. For the first time in a month, I was neither dizzy nor nauseous as I got out of bed. I could stand up straight in the shower and took great pleasure in the warm water streaming over my body. My mind continued to be clear, and once again I enjoyed the awareness of thoughts bouncing around in my head.

I was shocked when I finished my shower and looked at myself in the mirror. I must have seen myself in the bathroom mirror daily but with the disorientation my appearance hadn't registered in my brain. I'd lost easily twenty pounds: my clothes hung on me, and my eyes were sunken and dark. In the mirror I saw an emaciated version of what had been, only six months earlier, a fit, healthy, thirty-five-year-old. If I carried on like this, I knew I wouldn't see Christmas.

My stay at the motel brought relief from most of my symptoms. I was able to think clearly, sleep well, eat well, and get through the days without head swellings and nights without fevers and seizures. With clear thought, I could come to some realizations about my situation that would enable me to find ways of coping with my symptoms.

The fact that I was well when I was away from my house confirmed for me that my symptoms might well be caused by something in my environment rather than by an illness within me: my symptoms were a reaction to something external rather than an expression of internal disease. I realized that I was the only person who believed this and that I didn't have a lot of time to get the support and help that I needed. Without some kind of confirmation of my belief and a strategy for healing, I would soon be too ill to work out what was causing these symptoms. Once I reached a point where I was too weak to take care of myself, I would have to hand over the responsibility for my health to the doctors and let them treat my symptoms as an illness.

Restoring Balance

Though my parents did not believe that there was anything wrong with my house, they acknowledged that I believed it and were prepared to support me while I worked it out. They weren't convinced that I needed to see a psychiatrist. Their interpretation of the situation was that I had lost the balance in my life — but that it could be restored. To them, life's balance emanates from an active and focused mind, fresh air, nutritious food, time for contemplation, and individual space. Several things emerged from these beliefs that would help me on the road to recovery.

Like a true Swede, Dad believed in the restorative power of nature. He found himself a map, located the nearest lake, packed a picnic, and drove me up to it. He wanted me to "njuta av naturen" — to let nature make me feel good. The lake was in Barrie, a beautiful quiet place where I could sit and be at peace with nature. Here I could feel the strength of the elements: the clear air and the crystal water, the wind in my hair and the sun on my back. This place, where nature could wrap itself around me and make me feel good, was accessible. It was a sanctuary to which I could escape when the disorientation and head swellings made the world a very dark place.

My parents considered food, nutrition, and exercise another element of balance. Meals at my house had slipped from an orderly set table every night to: "Oh, is it that time already?" I couldn't even remember the last time I had been able to chew any food, or had felt hunger. They brought home-made food to me every day; never had Mum's meatloaf tasted so good, salad so crisp, and potatoes so creamy. My parents reminded me of the importance of eating and I realized that, whatever it took, I had to eat if I was going to regain my strength and to keep it. Food would soon become a measure of my success: for almost a year, I would survive from one meal to the next. If I could just eat breakfast, even if it had to be through a straw, then I would be all right until lunch; if I could just eat lunch, then I would be all right until supper; etc.

To give me something to think about other than myself, Mum paid for a set of piano lessons. I had always loved playing the piano and she felt a lesson each week would give me a focus. I managed to go to every lesson, though there were several where my right arm was too weak to play. But my teacher worked with my left hand and showed me how to add a base to any tune. In the short term, the lessons certainly helped to focus my attention and in the long term, as I got to the bottom of my troubles and regained the use of my right hand, the piano became an invaluable outlet.

So between the lake, food, and music my parents provided a framework in which to restore my psychological, spiritual, and physical balance. This restoration would take time but would ultimately help me cope with what lay ahead.

The Allergist

From the motel, I made an appointment to see another doctor. I presented him with the same set of symptoms that I had presented to the two previous doctors. This time, I emphasized that I was sure that I didn't feel the symptoms everywhere; they subsided when I left the house. I explained how I thought they were related to my environment. Where many had laughed, this doctor listened very attentively and patiently — and sent me for allergy testing.

My arms were pricked from elbow to pinky and the tests showed that I was allergic to everything. I had problems with trees, weeds, animals, dust, mold — you name it, I had become allergic to it. I tried to talk to the doctor who performed the test. I thought an allergist would be the perfect accredited professional to understand my symptoms and help me track down the cause, but he had little time for my story. He had never heard of symptoms like mine, nor had he ever heard of anyone becoming allergic to everything in such a short time. All he had to offer was some information on living with allergies and creating a sanctuary.

Creating a Sanctuary

The sanctuary would relieve my immune system from the allergens to which I had tested positive. I was to create this sanctuary by first choosing a room and then removing everything from it. I needed to carefully vacuum and wash the ceiling, floor, and walls, and to clean the windows and frames with a bleach solution to prevent or at least delay the renewed growth of mold.

With the room cleaned, I could bring back a bed and bedding that had been carefully washed and triple rinsed. I was not to keep anything in the cupboard or around the room, as any extras would attract and harbor dust. My sanctuary would need to be dusted and vacuumed daily. I needed to keep it separate from the dust and mold in the rest of the house by shutting the door and providing an alternate source of heat. Since we didn't have a forced air heating system, the electric baseboard heater in the room was fine.

The day I returned from the motel Mum, Dad, and I spent the day preparing the sanctuary. I was eager to try it. I felt so strong that my reasoning about my symptoms seemed almost absurd. I was anxious for any feedback that might confirm that I was on the right track. But that evening my world again came crashing down on me. Mum had prepared a lovely supper to celebrate my return to the house, but as I sat down to eat it, the head swellings came thick and fast. By the end of the meal my right hand had shriveled up and my jaws were tight and clunking.

I felt so disheartened that I went up into my new sanctuary, curled up into a ball, and sobbed. I could hear them all downstairs. They were all fine: they had spent three days in my house and felt nothing. "It just couldn't be," I heard them say. "It just couldn't be." I felt an unfathomable depth of despair as I listened to them talking. Maybe now my parents wouldn't believe me. We had worked so hard to prepare my sanctuary; just how much more could I expect them to do? How much time could they give me? And how much time would I need?

When I tried to express myself the next morning, the response was punctuated with questions such as: "What were you trying to say?", " You were saying?", and "What happened next?" My disorientation had returned full force and my ability to follow a thought through to its conclusion was again gone. I had constant head swellings; I had seizures when I went to bed and feverish sweat several times during the night; and I started the day with vomiting.

I continued to sleep in the sanctuary but ultimately realized that though it removed me from all the allergens to which I had tested positive, it had absolutely no impact on the symptoms for which I was trying to find a cause. A face full of dust or pollen would bring on the odd sneeze, but it had absolutely no impact on my head swellings, temperature sensitivity, nightly fevers, wasting arm, forgetfulness, etc.

I would later return to the theory of the sanctuary as a place where the burdens that undermined my natural defenses were removed. But at the time, this theory epitomized a way of thinking about allergies that just didn't work for me. It would have been one thing to avoid peanuts if I'd had a peanut allergy, or to find Ginger a new home had I been allergic to cats, but if I really was allergic to as many things as the allergy tests suggested, removing them all would leave me living in isolation. Life in a bubble was not a life I could accept. Though I continued with the sanctuary, I wanted to know what had suddenly undermined my natural defenses. I wanted to know why my symptoms persisted even when I removed the allergens the tests had shown me to be allergic to.

Purifying Air, Food, Fabric, and Water

The smell in my house still bothered me terribly; neither the extractor fan nor the dehumidifier had made a lasting impact. So, in the hope that an air purification specialist might be able to do something to control the smell, I approached several companies. None of them had any interest in domestic environments. They knew plenty about Sick Building Syndrome, but that was something associated with offices, not homes.

There was just one man, Bruce Small, who was willing to try to help me. He and his family had suffered terribly from sick house syndrome, and their symptoms had pursued them beyond their home. Eventually forced to move out of downtown Toronto, Bruce and his family built a "clean" house in the

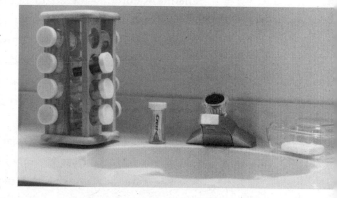

Spicing Up Your Toiletries. By storing essential toiletries and cosmetics in small glass containers like these ones in a spice rack, we can reduce our exposure — in terms of both time and quantity — to the chemicals they release into the air. **Photo**: *Angela Hobbs.*

suburbs. Indeed, the house was so clean that even the cupboards vented to the outside. Using his own sensitivities to chemicals and the knowledge that had enabled him to build his clean house, Bruce had set himself up as a consultant on Indoor Air Quality. Bruce was willing to share his solutions with me.

When Bruce pulled up in his beat-up old car, I was sure I was dealing with a charlatan out to milk me for every penny. He was wearing a well-worn shirt and jeans, had no equipment, and looked far from professional. But he was here, and so far he was the only person who had offered to help me. Other than my parents, he was the only person prepared to consider that my environment might be playing a role in my symptoms. He was my first connection to the world of sick houses and chemical sensitivities, and despite his somewhat unprofessional appearance, he had some proactive suggestions that might help to alleviate some of my symptoms.

Bruce spent the next two hours walking around my house sniffing. He agreed that there was a good chance that my symptoms were a reaction to something external rather than an expression of something internal. He considered that my house had a lot of odors that were creating a chemical concoction that my body was unable to tolerate, and this overload produced strange symptoms. He liked the sanctuary and advised me to try it for a bit longer. In order to lift the burdens on my body, giving it a chance to restore balance, I would need to try five simple methods of reducing the quantity of chemicals entering the air in my house. As I implemented each of his five suggestions, my reactions would confirm or deny my suspicions about the cause of my symptoms. He sat down and wrote out a plan.

It felt so good to be proactive rather than just to suffer the awful symptoms. I quite enjoyed taking my aluminum tape and sealing up holes. With each step that I implemented, my head cleared a little. Though not all of my symptoms were alleviated, I did gain control of my disorientation. By following Bruce's suggestions, I had lifted the burden on my body enough to enable me to think clearly in my home.

The time for my parents' departure loomed. They had come for a weekend and stayed two weeks. To say that they were torn at the prospect of leaving me would be an understatement. But if they were to qualify for health care in England, they had to go. In reality they had done what they could. They believed my ability to cope would improve and they knew that I knew they were only a phone call away.

Before they left, Dad filled every room but the sanctuary with spider plants and ferns. He had read about their tremendous capacity for removing toxins from the air. The downside to this newfound information, of course, is that it takes some eleven large spider plants to clear and maintain the air in just one room. And that's not taking into account any of the soil molds or pesticides that the plants may have been treated with.

With my parents gone and my disorientation under control, I resolved to look at my symptoms in relation to my environment. I continued to see doctors in the hope that there might be some help out there for me. And I began read. I scoured the stacks at the library looking for clues. I read everything I could find about allergies and Sick Building Syndrome — anything on healthy homes, natural healing, and wellness. If I thought there might be any chance of a clue, I searched. I also began to write: I kept a log of where my symptoms occurred, hoping that maybe, if I recorded everything I'd eaten or worn, everywhere I'd been, and what I'd been doing, then maybe, in time, a pattern would emerge. I firmly believed that the symptoms themselves held the answer.

> Did you know that three of the chemicals used in manufacturing synthetic fabrics have known side effects? Benzene is known to depress the central nervous system, causing headaches, dizziness, nausea, and convulsions. Ammonia causes burning sensations in the eyes, nose and throat, pain in the lungs, nausea, tearing, coughing, and an increased breathing rate. Ethylene glycol is that same poison we find in our windscreen washer fluid.[3]

The information I could find approached sensitivities from the top down. Each one, such as the elimination diet, approached sensitivities in terms of isolating and removing whatever was provoking the reaction. My symptoms were so varied that I was sure I would have to remove virtually everything from my environment if I followed this approach. It would give me no answers as to how I had suddenly developed so many sensitivities or what had undermined my immune system so rapidly. To answer these questions I needed more of a bottom-up approach — the type of approach I would use if my fish got sick, for instance.

Until coming to Newmarket I'd always kept fish. I knew that when they started staying at the bottom of the tank, there were a few things that I needed to do. I'd start by adjusting the environment — siphoning out an inch of water from the bottom of the tank and replacing it with chlorine-free water. I'd increase the oxygenation, check the food, temperature, and pH.

Five Ways to Clean the Air In Your House

1. **Eliminate Formaldehyde**: Formaldehyde is listed alongside PCBs, dioxin, and DDT as a Class B carcinogen by the US Environmental Protection Agency (EPA).[1] It is known to cause dizziness, coughing, and wheezing,[2] According to Bruce's plan, I was to diminish the amount of formaldehyde getting into my environment by sealing all exposed chipboard surfaces. Since the typical sealants — varnish and paint — had odors that would contribute to the overload on my body, I was to seal surfaces with aluminum tape. It took several days and many rolls of aluminum tape to cover all the chipboard surfaces in the house. We taped every chipboard or particleboard surface that was open to the air, and since I've always been a great IKEA shopper, that meant some serious taping. We got into cupboards and taped the holes, cracks, and dents. We taped under countertops and along shelf edges. Anywhere that there was a chance that formaldehyde could get out into the air got the aluminum treatment.

2. **Reduce Food Odors**: I was to decrease the level of odors by removing all foods that had an odor. I could store these either in containers made of glass or metal, or in the garage. I was not to use plastic containers because they smell. I went through my food cupboard; Bruce had actually ducked as he'd opened the doors because of his own sensitivities. Out came the brown sugar and the molasses, the peanut butter and the syrup. Out came the Jell-O and the children's cereal, and out came the spices.

3. **Store Cleaning Fluids Outside**: I was to store cleaning chemicals in the garage, not under the sink, and discard any that I wasn't using. Cleaning chemicals weren't really an issue for me since I've always balked at these odors; I've always avoided the cleaning aisle in the grocery store because I find the smell so strong. Even though the products are in containers, the chemicals leach into the air. So my Vim, laundry powder, and dish soap went out onto the garage shelves.

4. **Reconsider Cosmetics**: I had to go through my cosmetics, throw out anything I wasn't using, and store any others in sealed containers. I found it more difficult to implement this step — to actually deal with the cosmetics — than any of the other steps. It wasn't that I was any great hoarder of lipsticks or other cosmetics, but with the contaminants in my air so much reduced, I found I reacted badly to the smell of the cosmetics. The smell of soap, shampoo, and toothpaste were very strong to me — odors I'd never noticed before. I began airing my unperfumed soap in the garage for at least a month, as apparently a minimal amount of perfume is added even to unperfumed soap to mask the odors of the ingredients.

…continued on opposite page

Five Ways to Clean the Air In Your House – continued:

5. **Seal Off Basement**: The final step was to stop the air from the basement coming up into the house. Preventing the damp, moldy, basement air from penetrating through the house was easy. Fortunately (or so I thought so at the time), our electric baseboard heating meant no central fan was circulating the air in our house. Sealing off the basement meant keeping the basement door shut and stuffing and sealing the space around any pipes or wires that came up through the floor. However, once this step was complete, it became very obvious that at some point we would have to deal with the basement. Even with the basement windows left open, the mold was potent whenever we opened the basement door.

Only after I had exhausted every avenue of environmental modification would I turn to chemical remedies. Applying a similar approach to my own environment might help me unravel some of the answers to my questions.

Food

Since there didn't seem to be much more I could do with my air and my other symptoms didn't seem to have changed as the odors from formaldehyde, food, and cosmetics were lifted, I went on to look at the food I ate. At this point my symptoms included a wasting arm, temperature sensitivities, seizures, fevers, head swellings, forgetfulness, lack of balance, confusion, concentration difficulties, nausea, racing heartbeat, and occasionally blurred vision. By eliminating and reintroducing foods in related groups, I could establish any sensitivities to them — a procedure known as the elimination diet.

I began by blocking milk products. For a whole week I didn't consume anything containing milk or milk products. That meant cheese, butter, milk, cakes, chocolate, etc. After a week I reintroduced just a little and checked for reactions. There were none.

The following week I blocked wheat and wheat products: breads, gravies, pasta, cookies, cakes, cereals, etc. Again I reintroduced them gradually a week later, but when I checked for reactions, there were none.

The following week I eliminated yeast and anything containing yeast. I continued with this procedure until I had covered all the foods and additives normally in my diet. The only foods I didn't worry about, at that point, were the foods that would have required chewing. I could barely open my mouth and when I did, I was rewarded with a great big clunk and the problem of closing it again.

Fortunately I had already eliminated prepared foods since they had never done anything for me. I had always eaten foods either in their natural state, or so close to it that they were still recognizable.

The elimination diet brought me no closer to establishing connections between my symptoms and the environment. The exercise taught me to read the labels on food, and I learned all about disguised food additives. Though disappointed that I hadn't made any discoveries, I wasn't surprised. I'd always been interested in food and reacted against the idea of eating wheat three times a day — at breakfast as toast, at lunch as pizza, and at supper as pasta. I also tended to eat foods that were in season — often simply because they were cheaper. So my body wasn't always trying to digest the same foods day in day out, year in year out. I had learned to eat guavas, papayas, and sweet potatoes in Tanzania, rye bread and buttermilk in Sweden, herbal teas and sauerkraut in Germany, and fish and potatoes in England. I had combined these tastes with the result that, until this major upset, I had a great state of health that left me with boundless energy and only the rarest of colds. But that being said, something had certainly happened when I came to live in Newmarket that none of my healthy eating habits could contend with.

Fabric

Though eliminating and reading about food had been informative, it was the elimination of chemicals in my air that continued to have the greatest impact on my symptoms. With this in mind, I decided to look more closely at other chemicals in my environment — those in my clothes and in my water — to see what effect they had on my symptoms. So many of our fabrics are chemically based that I shouldn't have been surprised by my findings. As I had done with food, I eliminated and reintroduced one fabric at a time. During my first week I wore only well-worn, washed, and triple-rinsed cotton — underwear included. The second week I added a polyester sweatshirt equally well washed and rinsed but not as well worn. Within five minutes my head was spinning and the sweatshirt was off. I tried again three days later with a polyester sweater, and again couldn't wait to get it off.

If we think back to that organic chemistry we studied in school, it is hardly surprising that these fabrics caused a reaction. Making synthetic fibers is much the same as making goop! We start out with liquids — chemicals like benzene, ammonia, ethylene glycol, sulfuric acid hexamethylenediamine, hydroxylamine, terephthalic acid, propylene, etc. Mix them together and add a little heat for good measure. The resulting goop is then spun into a fiber and woven into material.

Between each attempt at wearing a fabric other than my well-washed and triple-rinsed cottons, I would allow three days. Each time I reintroduced polyester I was overcome with dizziness, even when the garment label claimed a minimal percentage. I eventually got rid of all my polyester or polyester-mix clothes, sheets, blankets, etc. My reaction to rayon and acrylic was similar though not as severe, possibly because of the cellulose content. In time I was able to reintroduce rayon and some acrylic, but only if it was well worn, well washed, and well rinsed.

Water

Drinking Water

The final aspect of my environment that required consideration was water. I consumed vast quantities of tap water, preferring it to sweetened drinks and sodas. Maybe the distasteful, heavily chlorinated water in my house was causing my symptoms. I tracked down a source of purified water at a nearby water store. Stories about chemicals in plastic migrating into bottled water left me with little interest in the water bottles that line the grocery store shelves. At the water store, I filled my own bottle with water purified by reverse osmosis and passed through a charcoal filter. At first I used a glass bottle but eventually began to use the blue plastic bottle, small enough that I could refill it daily, but light enough to deal with.

When I first brought the plastic bottle home, I could taste the plastic in the water. For the first month I didn't find the water the least bit palatable and so I continued with my glass bottle while I soaked the plastic taste out of the plastic bottle. Every day I would fill the plastic bottle with water and leave it to stand in a warm place. The following day, I would empty it and then refill it with fresh water. After about a month, the plastic taste was gone and I began using it for my reverse osmosis water.

Did you know that chlorine is used to disinfect the water in 90 percent of North American homes? Chlorine turns your hair green, rots bathing suits, and kills tropical fish. It was used as a poison gas in World War I, yet it is only rarely removed from water before distribution. In ordinary tap water, chlorine combines with organic compounds creating highly toxic chloro-organic compounds that may be linked to cancer.[4]

Bathing Water

Now that I had dealt with the water going into my body, I needed to deal with the water outside my body. Our skin is the largest sense organ in our bodies and I was subjecting mine on a daily basis to assaults by chlorine and a whole host of other chemicals and stuff. Indeed there is so much stuff in Newmarket's water that, according to a plumber who installed my water softener, an inert iron compound has to be added just to stop the pipes from clogging! Purifying all the water coming into my house by reverse osmosis seemed unnecessary. What I could do was filter out some of the gunk. In order to do this, I bought a water softener and added charcoal to the resin base. The charcoal would filter out a lot of the chlorine in the water and the resin would do its best with the rest.

Cleaning my water had a tremendous impact on my disorientation, and anything that diminished my disorientation made me feel stronger and more able to cope. I could hold my own with Lawrence and Joan, and I could cope with the many different diagnoses by the doctors in my life.

With my water, air, clothing and food so purged of chemicals, I seemed to be more sensitive to them than ever. I could smell the toothpaste in the upstairs bathroom from the living room when the children forgot to put it back in the garage. I had become so sensitive to chlorine that I couldn't even take a shortcut across the field at the local sports complex — yet I'd always been an avid swimmer. And the odd waft of steam from the clothes dryer carried into my house on a gentle breeze would send me running for cover.

More Symptoms, Doctors and Diagnoses

My efforts to use elimination as a means of establishing what it was about my environment that had undermined my immune system, leaving me allergic to everything and experiencing symptoms that didn't correlate to the diagnosed allergens, had come to an end. The diligent examination of my air, food, clothing, and water had not produced the connections I'd hoped for. I was clearly better off without the chemicals, but I was still very unwell. I had been in my house for eight months and I had been sick and semi-dysfunctional for six. I was still having almost continuous head swellings. I was still having seizures and fevers at night. I was still on an emotional roller coaster. And I still had this awful tingling, shriveling hand. I was still suffering, still frightened, and still not getting any better. I was now in a situation where I could no longer blame my environment for my illness. I had tried so hard to take responsibility for my own health. I had really believed that my symptoms were a reaction to something in my environment rather than an expression of something from within. A terrible feeling of defeat set in as I began drawing the conclusion that I must have been wrong.

As if I hadn't suffered enough, I now began to get stabbing pains in my neck. These pains were fierce and came very suddenly with no warning. I absolutely could not deal with or learn to live with this kind of pain, so I went off to see another doctor. This doctor suspected a brain tumor. Of course, he couldn't give me a final diagnosis until I had undergone a CAT scan, but he was pretty sure that it would be worth doing.

The rug had been pulled from under me. Was this possible? Had this been what was wrong all along? Surely there were a whole host of other symptoms that went with brain tumors and where were they? What happened to this brain tumor when I was in the motel and at Betty's? Why wasn't I having headaches? I was seriously disturbed by this latest diagnosis, but I wasn't about to do anything without a second opinion.

So off I went to yet another doctor. Presented with the same set of symptoms, this doctor suspected multiple sclerosis. Again, without tests she couldn't be sure, but she felt an MRI would be worth doing and she would get me onto the waiting list. Again, I insisted on a second opinion and went off to another doctor. Presented with the same symptoms, this time the doctor suspected Chronic Fatigue Syndrome.

In the space of two weeks I had seen three doctors and presented them with exactly the same set of symptoms in the hope of getting a consistent diagnosis. I had come away with three different diagnoses of three very serious illnesses and I was well and truly scared and bewildered. I agreed to see a neurologist and undergo both the MRI and the CAT scan. I hoped that maybe they would reveal something treatable or removable. The lack of consensus between the doctors regarding the cause of my symptoms left me very skeptical of their diagnoses. I would be much more comfortable accepting a diagnosis and treatment if two doctors agreed. How could I trust a doctor who seemed more bewildered than I was, or who laughed at my suspicions that my symptoms might be related to my environment. As it was, I had more answers than I knew what to do with, and I had more questions than I would ever have time to ask.

I tried hard to find encouragement where I could in my quest for time. If I could stop myself getting any worse, then maybe I would come across a piece of information that would make sense out of this conundrum. There were basically two ways I had of doing this: meals and balance. If I could eat breakfast, I'd be all right until lunch, and if I could eat lunch, I'd get through to supper. The other measure of success was to stand in an empty space and shut my eyes. If I could lift a leg and hold my balance for fifteen seconds, I was doing well. If, on the other hand, I couldn't get past two seconds without tumbling, it was time for me to take a break from my house and go for a walk. If a walk didn't increase my balance time, I would head up to Barrie and the lake. Invariably a trip to the lake would restore me to an easy fifteen-second balance and a walk in a local park could usually get me back up to seven. Later, as I struggled my way back to health, these little measures of success became my yardstick.

Money played a huge role in my reliance on conventional medicine and myself. Naturopathic medicine is not covered by health care in Ontario. The ridicule that my suspicions evoked from everyone around me made me wary of spending family money on what my husband considered my little obsession. If I were going to spend money I had to be sure that the person I was paying would have some answers. But if there was a chance that they had some answers for me, it might be a road worth traveling.

The focus of naturopathic medicine on man's interaction with his environment made it a definite point of curiosity for me. In reality however, it seemed that the approach of many of the naturopaths I called didn't differ significantly from that of conventional medicine. I went to many of the free talks that were being given by these practitioners of alternative medicine. I learned a lot about alternative medicine, about tinctures and supplements, the immune system, exercise, balancing the body and mind, and generally about natural health. I also called several naturopaths to get an idea of their individual understanding and approach to health. At every opportunity I would briefly describe my symptoms and the work I had done on elimination and ask where they would start. Virtually all of them would start with a hefty consultation fee, followed by allergy testing, and then recommendations for food and vitamin supplements.

It seemed to me that naturopaths were no more interested in listening to my approach than the doctors of conventional medicine had been. If I was going to take medicine at all, then I had more faith in conventional medicine than in herbal potions. But fundamentally, I wasn't looking for medicine. I didn't want to take anything; I wanted to remove whatever it was that was causing my symptoms. As I struggled with my questions Christmas approached.

I came out of the holidays weak and ready to give up. My mother-in-law had joined us from England for the celebration. I vaguely remember the electric baseboard heating being on all the time, the turkey cooking all day, the air being full of perfume, and all the windows being closed. After two weeks of these circumstances, I barely had the strength to get myself out of the house.

The thought that the New Year would hold an MRI and a CAT scan was almost a relief. There would finally be an explanation of what was wrong with me. I would discover why I didn't have symptoms by the lake in Barrie, or, for that matter, anywhere north of Bradford. Radiation and drugs would replace my pure world. What chance would I have against the pharmaceutical world if I couldn't even tolerate the chemicals in my house? But there was just no more I could do.

Weak and defeated, I prepared to give up the fight, but there was just one more lecture that I wanted to go to — a talk on natural health by a chiropractor, a talk at which the opening words were: "Did you know that at any given time, any membrane in the body can react to any allergen?"

A small group of people had gathered in the library for this public lecture that would lay the foundation for my recovery. The lecturer — a tall, lean, very healthy looking doctor — began by answering the question on the tip of all our tongues: why was a chiropractor giving a lecture on natural health? He explained that his introduction to natural health had come through his daughter, who had suffered from a variety of symptoms that conventional medicine seemed unable to relieve. Determined to help his daughter, this chiropractor searched high and low for answers — a search that had led him to an understanding of his daughter's symptoms in relation to the environment that he and his wife had created for her.

When his talk was over, this doctor — whose name, unfortunately, has now been lost to me in a sea of doctors' names — responded to the concerns of his audience. The questions being asked and the symptoms being described seemed no stranger than my own, so I mustered up the courage to ask the questions and describe the symptoms that had made so many doctors laugh. This doctor listened without ridicule to my story and my queries about the possibility of environmental causes. When I was finished, he suggested that since I had worked through every other aspect of my environment, I might consider the effect of electricity.

After the discouragement I had faced, it was an enormous relief to have someone acknowledge that my symptoms could be connected to my environment. A doctor, someone who ought to know, had agreed that it was possible that my symptoms were a reaction to an external stimulus rather than the expression of internal disease.

Based on the premise that "at any given time, any membrane in the body can react to any allergen," this doctor suspected that electricity might be causing a membrane in my head to swell. Though the most common membranes to react to allergens are those in the nose and lungs, any membrane in the body can swell. From my description, this doctor surmised certain facts regarding my environment:

- I lived in a high-density housing development with baseboard heating;
- there was a stream under my house; and
- I lived near a microwave dish or a power station.

Was this really possible? Was it the oven that had caused my unbearable symptoms on Christmas day, not just the smell of turkey and perfume? Was it the fluorescent light above my head that made washing the dishes so stressful and not just the detergent? Was it the microwave that caused the stabbing pains in my neck?

I left the talk full of more questions. How would Lawrence react? He'd been so good about my efforts to find a connection. Each day he would come home to find another little something banished to the garage shelf. He couldn't brush his teeth or put on his dry-cleaned suit without making a trip to the garage. And even an innocent look at the newspaper required a trip to the garage. And now I was going to ask him to believe this! Would he help me pursue this new lead, or would I have to move out? Would this be the final straw? Would it cost me my children?

3

Coming to Terms with Electricity

THE POSSIBILITY THAT ELECTRICITY MIGHT BE THE FACTOR IN MY ENVIRONMENT that was causing my difficulties was awfully difficult to accept. While part of me reacted with relief that there might still be hope, another part found it incredible. Electricity was something clean, not dirty like oil and gas. It had no odor and it was invisible. Hadn't my father had an electric heating system custom designed when he built his house in gas-heated England, precisely because electricity was so clean that he was prepared to go to the added expense? In all my life I had never heard of electricity being anything but clean, desirable, healthy, and good. After thirty-five years of taking this pollution-free energy for granted, how was I to persuade my brain that it might hold some answers for me? Though it seemed almost absurd that electricity could be causing my symptoms, my alternative was to accept the diagnoses and treatment of conventional medicine. What choice did I really have?

Until now Lawrence had pretty much stayed on the sidelines watching my health deteriorate. I'd reported each of the doctors' suspicions and he was as confused as I was with such an array of diagnoses. In the meantime he did what he could. He would take me up to the lake in Barrie whenever I asked him to, and tried not to say too much about the state of the house. But fundamentally he still thought I needed to see a psychiatrist. There had always been quick-fix solutions to our previous problems and it was intensely frustrating that this situation didn't have one. Though we felt ill-equipped to deal with this situation, we were probably better equipped than most. I, after all, had the symptoms in my body, and Lawrence had trained as an air traffic engineer. He had an understanding of electricity and radio waves that I would be able to tap into to find my answers. Lawrence had found my previous attacks on the environment almost as absurd as the doctors did, but now that I was talking about something he could understand, he was prepared to discuss the possibilities and become part of the solution.

One of the most obvious differences between the environment by the lake in Barrie, where I felt good, and the environment at home, where I felt awful, was the level of electricity. At home I was in a high density, baseboard-heated housing development with every electrical convenience imaginable. In my favorite spot in Barrie, there were a few street lamps, a huge expanse of calm water, no houses, and no electrical conveniences. The overall amount of electricity in the two environments was significantly different.

The disparity between these two environments — and my symptoms in them — gave weight to the possibility of electricity being a factor in my ill health. But if, indeed, electricity was involved, just what could I do about it? I wasn't dealing with a tangible, visible foe here, as had been in the case of foods, fabrics, water, and odors. If this latest hypothesis were true, then first proving it and then dealing with it were well beyond the scope of my experience. At school I had always just scraped a passing mark in science; my degree was in Scandinavian Studies, and my teaching had been limited to children under twelve. I was absolutely not the material of which rocket scientists and doctors are made. At this point, it probably would have been easier to accept the diagnosis of conventional medicine and give up the fight. But as I looked into the eyes of my boys, my beautiful boys whom I had brought into this world against so many odds, I knew I had to fight until I had exhausted all my options.

Though I could never be a scientist or a neurosurgeon, I did have something that they didn't have: I had the head and arm in which the symptoms were taking place. I wasn't looking for a PhD; I just wanted to understand what it was about my environment that was doing this to me — and how I could make it stop.

If I could follow the reactions of my body and inform myself about the basics of electricity, then maybe I could find some answers. As with each of my attacks on the environment, I began by working my way through the library stacks. I read anything that might give me a better understanding of electricity. I learned about fuses and fuse boxes, distribution centers, electric coils, electric fields, magnetic fields, frequencies, wavelengths and voltages. Electricity ceased to be something that just happened when I flicked the switch and became a series of invisible waves permeating the air around me.

Ever the arts graduate, I had to find parallels in my experience for everything I read about electricity. The only way I could make sense of the information I was reading and gain an understanding of this invisible, intangible foe was by visualizing it. My first vision was of a whole army of little electrons (complete with red suits) marching down wires. Some of these wires were visible, some were underground, and some were in the walls. As the little red suits marched down the wires, they created fields of energy in the air. The more tightly packed they were, the more intense was the energy field they created in the air around them.

Though I was gaining an understanding of electricity, I was still far from seeing how it could be affecting me. With my previous attacks on the environment, I had been able to eliminate and reintroduce things one by one. With electricity I would not be able to use this technique — I couldn't eliminate electricity from my environment. Even if I accepted the possibility that electricity was causing my symptoms, what could I do about it?

The Log

The only way I could see of finding connections between electricity and my symptoms was to add another dimension to my already detailed log. At this point I was suffering from head swellings, a wasting arm, forgetfulness, stabbing pains in my neck, temperature sensitivity, painful jaws, inappropriate laughing and crying, poor balance, and seizures and fevers at night. Each time I had one of my symptoms, I would record not only what I had eaten, where I had been, what I was wearing, and the time of day, etc. — now I would also draw my position in the room and record the appliances that were on at the time. I hoped that in doing this I would eventually build up a pattern that would give me some clues.

It didn't take long before I knew I was on to something. Once I began associating my symptoms with appliances being turned on, it was obvious that there was a connection. The head swellings would come thick and fast whenever the fluorescent light in the kitchen or laundry room was on. As soon as the fluorescent light was turned off, the swellings would gradually slow and then stop. It didn't matter where I was in the house: I didn't need to be in the kitchen or the laundry room to feel the head swellings. From anywhere in the house I could tell when someone had inadvertently turned on a fluorescent light. Of course, I had been taught that it is more energy efficient to leave fluorescent lights on during the day than to be constantly turning them on and off. Consequently, the fluorescent lights in the kitchen and basement had been left on all day. At night, I would turn them off just before I went to bed. As I kept my log, it became very clear that my head swellings were almost wholly related to the fluorescent lights.

Within a week I had control of my head swellings. I was so elated that I had finally, after several weeks of up to seventy head swellings a day, found a way to make them stop. I could finally leave my corner where I had spent so many days curled up, sobbing, and holding my head, just begging the head swellings to stop.

My efforts to connect my environment and my symptoms were beginning to pay off. I now had ways of controlling both my disorientation and my head swellings. I limited my disorientation by keeping my air, clothes, and water free of chemicals, and limited my head swellings by using alternatives to fluorescent lights. After many long months of suffering I had finally reached a turning point. Gaining control of my two most debilitating symptoms gave me a tremendous feeling of empowerment and the hope that I would eventually find a way of eliminating all of my symptoms.

I continued to keep a log of my position and appliances that were turned on in the hope of finding a way of alleviating my nausea, fevers, seizures, painful jaws, useless arm, and emotional roller coaster. But though I was diligent, the only other obvious connection I could establish was that the stabbing pains in my neck would come when the microwave and stove were on at the same time. For now, I would have to content myself with escaping my other symptoms by leaving the house as much as possible and spending large amounts of time by the lake in Barrie. Lawrence began to indulge me with frequent trips to Muskoka and regular nights at motels — indulgences that we could ill afford but my health was at stake and I was so much stronger after each trip and so much more functional that it seemed the best thing we could do.

Whenever we returned to the house after a stay at the motel, my symptoms would be relatively mild until I went to bed. Comparing the two environments, I wondered just what role a good night's sleep was having on my symptoms and my ability to cope with them. It seemed to me that the feverless, seizure-free, sound sleep that I got at the motel might be playing a role in my increased strength. Conversely, the disturbed sleep that I got at home might be playing a role in taking this strength away. My focus now became finding a way of getting a good night's sleep at home.

The chiropractor who had alerted me to the effects of electricity had suggested that the stream under my house might be one of the factors adding to the EMFs in my house. My reading had suggested that the stream contributed by reflecting the EMFs back into the house rather than allowing them to follow their natural course into the ground. With this information, we decided that if we could block the reflection, we might be able to reduce the ambient level of electricity around me. In order to create a barrier, we built the equivalent of a flat Faraday's cage. We soldered together two pieces of mesh about five feet square and then earthed (grounded) them through the window to the ground outside. This was then covered with a carpet and at night I would roll my bedding out onto the carpet and sleep. Unfortunately, after five nights on the Faraday's cage I was no better than I had been upstairs in the guest room. I still woke up vomiting and went to bed with seizures and fevers.

The Radio

Not to be deterred, I decided to try to use the radio to find a place to sleep. I had often noticed that the car radio fuzzed as we approached traffic lights and power lines. The static on the radio often coincided with a mounting pressure in my head and a racing of my heart. Of course, this could be a figment of my imagination, but it seemed to me that if power lines could make the radio fuzz then maybe the electricity in my house would make it fuzz, too. I had nothing to lose by being wrong and if I was right, then the radio had the potential to become a tool.

Armed with a radio, I began to explore the possibilities. I had to play with the radio for quite a while before I could see just how I would be able to use it. I'd walk around each room, getting increasingly frustrated at the way the sound seemed to constantly fuzz and fade depending on the way I held it. Slowly I realized that if I found a channel that fuzzed at the same time that pressure began to build in my head, then maybe I would be on to something. It took quite some doing, and I had to start from scratch several times, but I eventually found a channel that consistently fuzzed at the same time that pressure built in my head.

My hope now was that I would be able to use the fuzzing from the radio to locate a place in my house where I could sleep without my night-time symptoms. But before I could trust that the radio was reliable, I wanted to repeat my experiment at Joan's house. I'd spent enough time at her house to know where the places were that I felt a pressure building in my head. I calibrated the radio in Joan's house using the fuzzing in the spots where I was uncomfortable. As I had at home, I then moved the radio to check the spots where I'd felt pressure and sure enough the radio picked up the same spots as I did. What was most curious though was that I could walk through Joan's house with minimal interference to this channel other than the spots that I had already identified. However, when I walked through my own house, there were very few places that didn't get interference and of them only two were at sleeping height.

Two of my neighbors were happy to let me walk through their houses with my radio; my preoccupation was quite the subject of amusement as they sat on the green transformer boxes outside their houses and drank coffee. According to the radio, neither Tess' nor Laura's house had any fewer clear spots than mine did.

Elated at the prospect of having found a tool, I began to test the beds by combing the bedrooms at sleeping level inch by inch with the radio. I was looking for places where the radio at my confirmed spot on the dial didn't fuzz. These were places that I would consider "clean." As it turned out, Lawrence had been sleeping in one of these clean spots all this time. My children, whom I'd tried so hard to keep safe, were sleeping in the worst places of all! Richard and Christopher's pillows were virtually directly above the electrical service panel. The other clean spot was in the sanctuary, but not where I had had my head.

I was terribly eager to try this spot now and had Lawrence move my bed so that my head would be positioned right in the middle of this area. As with the Faraday's cage, I would give this spot five nights before I rushed to any conclusions. But after five nights of peaceful, restful sleep with no fevers, and waking, not with a clear head, but certainly without nausea, there was only one conclusion to be drawn. I had found a way of sleeping in my house with relative comfort. The seizures remained along with the tingling useless arm, but the inappropriate laughing and crying gradually became appropriate again.

The great advances that I had made since being introduced to the concept of electricity as an allergen made it clear that electricity was indeed playing a large role in the symptoms that I had been suffering.

With my discovery of a clear spot where I could sleep in relative comfort, all my symptoms became much milder. They were still uncomfortable, but after what I'd been through, I could live with them. The problem now became the health of the rest of my family. I began to notice just how thin and quiet Christopher had become. He had a really persistent cough that had been treated repeatedly with antibiotics. Much like my symptoms, though, his cough hadn't come to the motels with him — and that was the only place that I had been coherent enough to take care of him. He coughed and complained of earaches when we were at home, but when we were in motels or away from home elsewhere, he was all right. Much as I loved my children, I had been too sick to do anything but go through the motions of being a mother and not a very good one at that.

In the hopes that Christopher's health might take a turn for the better given similar sleep to myself, I asked Lawrence to trade beds with him. Chris was soon looking stronger. His silence still filled the air but he was eating well and his constant coughing at night stopped. Lawrence, on the other hand, developed bronchitis within a week. For the first time in his life, he had to take time off work and while he was home, the bronchitis quickly spread deeper into his lungs and he ended up with pneumonia.

Lawrence's pneumonia marked a real turning point in the life of our family. I was really unwilling to leave my new sleeping place, unless it was for the motel. I was adamant that Christopher should stay in the other clear sleeping spot that Lawrence had given up. That, though, meant that Lawrence had to continue sleeping where he was or find an alternative place without disturbing either Chris or myself. After a month, Lawrence was still sick; the pneumonia continued to linger and he returned to the doctor for ever-stronger doses of antibiotics. Spending so much time at home, Lawrence began to see his environment in a different light. For the first time, he saw that despite all my efforts at modifying my environment, I still spent most of the day like a zombie. He began to suspect that maybe our environment had been affecting Christopher and that now it was affecting him, too. Eventually, in desperation, he agreed that we needed to go and stay at the motel until he got better.

After ten months of watching me sink into symptoms no one could understand, Lawrence agreed that there was something intrinsically wrong with our environment. There was something with which we were incompatible — something that had attacked me first, and which he now was beginning to believe might attack all of us. If we didn't take control of our situation, there was a chance that the health of each member of our family would be compromised.

It gradually became very clear that we were going to have to change our environment. We were going to have to sell our house and move again. But before we could contemplate this, there were some questions we needed to answer.

Firstly, if electricity was really causing my symptoms, then why wasn't everyone else sick, too? Surely little Richard, who'd been born three months early, should have been the first to get sick. Yet of all of us, he was probably the healthiest. Only much later would I consider that his health might have been greatly helped by his nightly wanderings. Unlike Chris, who slept deeply on his pillow virtually above the electrical panel, Richard spent most of his nights moving from bed to bed around the house. More often than not he ended up snuggled close to Lawrence in that other clean spot. Could it be that the two months Richard spent in the incubator, recently shown to have an average magnetic field of 10 milligauss,[1] had already sensitized him to electricity and that this little three-year-old had used his intuition to find a clean spot? We had always thought he was looking for the physical contact he'd missed in his incubator.

Sick Neighborhood Syndrome?

Given the chiropractor's premise that "at any given time, any membrane in the body can swell in response to any allergen," we wondered if maybe the pneumonia, migraines, and sinus problems that Lawrence had developed since moving to Newmarket were also a result of the EMFs in the community. Christopher had been off school for a total of forty days and had been on seven different doses of antibiotics in nine months for bronchitis, strep throat, tonsillitis, and earaches. Could it be that these were caused by these same EMFs? As I'd gained strength, I had begun volunteering in Christopher's class and had been struck by the general state of health of the children. In my experience as a teacher, I had only once come across a child with an inhaler for asthma. In this class there were seven children who used inhalers every four hours and four others who used inhalers daily. Three children carried anaphylactic shock needles for allergies and on any given day there were at least five children with heavy bronchial coughs. Of the remainder there were endless sniffling noses and an acute lack of attention to the task at hand. Initially I had thought that Christopher had got his infections from his classmates. But now I began to wonder if electricity was playing a role in both his and his classmates' ill health.

Looking up and down the street, I realized we had neighbors who had had multiple miscarriages and others who suffered with psoriasis, migraines, depression, multiple sclerosis, leukemia, allergies, and asthma, asthma, and more asthma. I was undoubtedly living in a community of the sickest people I had ever met. Could it be that electricity was the factor that was making the fundamental difference?

The general poor health of my neighbors began setting off alarm bells. Could it be that electricity was creating the substantial difference between this community and the other communities in which I had lived? Was that why it had been so difficult to understand what was wrong or different about this environment? As we looked around our neighborhood and our house, we realized that the chiropractor's suspicions of electric baseboard heating, a stream under the house, and proximity to a microwave dish and power station were all accurate and, in time, we would come to realize the implications. If we thought about the ambient level of electricity in our neighborhood, there were several factors that would cause it to be higher than in others:

- the housing development was dense — we were all on 40-foot lots;
- the development had been built at a time when all-electric homes were the fashion;
- each of these all-electric homes required 200-ampere service instead of the more usual 100-amp service;
- the high water table prevented the passage of electric fields into the ground — instead, it acted as a reflector returning the fields back into our living space;
- there was a microwave relay dish staring at us from the top of a nearby apartment building;
- the electricity substation was two blocks away.

As with most subdevelopments, ours was served by the big-green-box type of transformers stationed every five or six houses. Their purpose was to reduce the voltage and increase the current from underground cables before it went into the houses. We assumed that the underground cables ran in straight lines between the boxes thereby creating a high current grid under the entire neighborhood. Above our heads along every road there were power lines running between other communities and the local substation, which

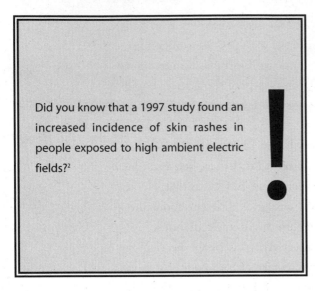

Did you know that a 1997 study found an increased incidence of skin rashes in people exposed to high ambient electric fields?[2]

essentially meant that this power grid was within a huge coil. It seemed to us that, taking all of this into consideration, the 60 Hz electrical fields in and around our house had to be many times that of the average neighborhood.

It seemed to us that there was a good chance that the high levels of electricity were affecting the whole community, but that virtually everyone was unwilling to consider it as a factor. Maybe some of the residents had never known anything else. Maybe they'd been living there for such a long time that they hadn't noticed the gradual increase in use of electricity as more and more peripheral communities sprang up. I began thinking about all the little bits of information that my interaction with the people in my community had provided. Even allowing for the possibility that I would have steered the conversations toward symptoms, following the age-old saying that "misery loves company," there was a definite trend toward the thinking that ailments were an expression of an internal illness or inadequacy rather than a reaction to an external stimulus.

Tess

One of my neighbors with psoriasis had been battling the sores and rashes on her skin for years. She single-handedly kept Newmarket's naturopaths employed! Each time she finished an elimination diet, there was another food that she had become allergic to. Each time she put herself through a cleansing therapy, she came out more sensitive to foods than she had been when she began.

What I found most interesting about my neighbor was that whenever she went away to visit family she came home without any psoriasis. Within three or four days she was breaking out from head to toe. Yet, despite the fact that she had filled her holiday with pizza and junk food and had had no problems with her psoriasis, she maintained that the psoriasis that appeared when she got home was the response of her body to the build-up of junk food. Indeed, much of the time she explained away her symptoms as the accumulation of toxins in her body. So why did they only accumulate when she was in Newmarket? How was it that she could spend one week away and return to a major outbreak of psoriasis, or she could spend four weeks away without the psoriasis and return to an almost immediate outbreak? If the build-up of toxins from the junk food was single-handedly causing the psoriasis, then why wasn't there a build-up anywhere else?

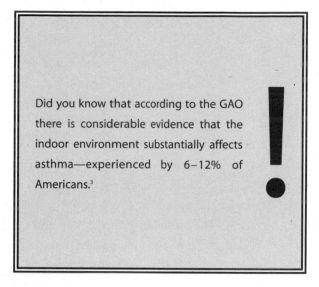

Did you know that according to the GAO there is considerable evidence that the indoor environment substantially affects asthma—experienced by 6–12% of Americans.[3]

Laura

During the time I spent in Newmarket, one of my other neighbors developed asthma. In her case it didn't run in the family, and she had never had any problems with breathing in the past. She and her family had moved to our development in Newmarket just months before we did. Like us, they found themselves suffering from more bouts of colds, flu, earaches, and bronchitis than they had ever known before. But they put the family's sudden ill health down to their increasing age (they were in their late thirties) and the cold winter. To Laura, asthma was just something that unlucky people got. Nothing causes it and nothing takes it away; the best you can hope for is that you might control it with medication or grow out of it.

Whichever way I turned up or down the street, virtually every person living in the development had some sickness to report. There was something here — and it was something with which we were incompatible and which we were powerless to control. Had my symptoms been in my leg, my skin, or my stomach I might have been tempted to explain them away as the weather or the food or anxiety, too. But my symptoms were in my head; they had all developed since moving into this neighborhood — and they very clearly indicated that there were places outside this environment where they were willing to leave me alone. The relief from my symptoms was virtually immediate when I was outside this environment. Unlike psoriasis, it didn't take two days to clear up. I think I had a huge advantage over my neighbors in that the relief to my symptoms was so immediate. Their connection to my environment was virtually unmistakable once I had the clarity of thought and the conviction to make the connection.

Lawrence's pneumonia really marked a turning point in my fight for answers. Our environment became his priority. For the first time since moving to Newmarket, he took a good long look at what was going on. The saga had continued for ten long months and I had found no long-term answers. During that time I had changed everything in my house except its physical location. I had dealt with the mold in the basement, an electrician had checked the wiring, and the new finishes had had a year to offgas — overall my house was probably safer than many of the houses in the community. Had my symptoms been limited to my house, I would have had some serious qualms about selling it, but it was quite clear to me that since I had to leave the whole area to get any relief, the house itself was not the problem. The time had come for us to seriously consider selling our house and move. We had to accept that we were incompatible with our environment. Despite the financial difficulty that the real estate commission would create for us and despite the possibility that I might be wrong, my only chance to regain my health lay in locating a compatible environment.

While we waited for our house to sell, the four of us doubled up in the two clear spots that I had found. This was the first month in our house where nobody got sick all month. Though my own symptoms were only just bearable, they were far better than they had been. There were some nights, usually wet rainy ones, when the clear spots became fuzzy. I would bend down to kiss the boys and feel that pressure building in my head. Convinced that my children were not safe, Lawrence and I would bundle them up into the car and head for our motel. For the duration of this month we worked on the theory that if we could sleep in the places that didn't have EMFs, we would be able to get through the next day without sickness. If we slept in the areas where the EMFs were high, we would return to, or remain in the familiar pattern of symptoms that had permeated the whole family and were compromising our health. Whether or not this was the way to go about it, it was what we felt we could do and it left us feeling proactive rather than beaten.

At the end of May our house was sold. The day the offer firmed up, I took my children out of school and headed for my parents' holiday home in Maine. We would spend the next eight weeks in their care while Lawrence rented a place in Barrie and we looked at our future.

In Search of a Compatible Environment

On the Move Again...

DURING THE YEAR THAT FOLLOWED THE MOVE FROM MY HOUSE IN NEWMARKET, I learned a lot about the connection between my environment and my symptoms. My initial hope — that moving would in itself return me to the state of health I had enjoyed before Newmarket — was somewhat unrealistic. Regardless of how carefully the environment was chosen, I would ultimately have to learn how to tailor my environment to suit myself. Each of three new environments initially seemed more comfortable, but gradually my symptoms crept back. I was left bewildered and increasingly convinced that the diagnosis of conventional medicine might be right. Whereas about thirty doctors were sure my symptoms were an expression of internal disease, only I and the chiropractor who suggested electricity entertained the thought that my symptoms were a reaction to an external stimulus. The odds seemed heavily stacked against me, and other than my symptoms and suspicions I had no pre-set path to follow, no back-up, and no proof. With every decision that we made the possibility that I might be wrong was factored in — from shortening Lawrence's commute to lighten his load if he became a single parent, to purchasing a bungalow that would accommodate a wheelchair.

Bridgton, Maine

The first of my comfortable environments was provided by my parents' summerhouse in Maine. Both chemically and electromagnetically, it was relatively clean. It was situated on a huge plot of land bordered by a park, a lake, a sawmill, and one neighbor. One small power line brought electricity to the house from the distribution line along the main road some two hundred feet away. Chemically, the house was well aged with most of the interior finishings being over ten years old. There was no new smell, no musty odor, and no dust that greeted you when you opened the door. Mum was determined that I should have no part in the household duties of cooking, cleaning, and laundry and she was happiest when I was sitting by the lake watching my children swim. I doubt that I could have found a more restorative environment than this. There was balance, love, and harmony with nature, clean air, and low EMFs. If I couldn't be well here, then there wasn't much chance for me. For the first six weeks in my parents' care I went from strength to strength. I even managed to get involved in the town's day camp, helping the children with crafts and activities before they went off for their afternoon swim in Highland Lake.

But for the last two weeks of my stay, my symptoms gradually began to return. At first I was dizzy in the morning, my right arm weakened, and gradually I started bumping into things as my balance began to deteriorate again. Both of my brothers had come to Bridgton with their families, one from Wales and the other from Washington. In the light of the gradual return of my symptoms, the family reunion seemed more poignant to me. If the diagnoses of conventional medicine were right, this might be the last time I would know who these people were; the chances that my mind would still be intact just months ahead were slim. That possibility hung over me like a dark cloud. As I watched my little nieces and nephews playing in the water with my own children, seven in all, a terrible feeling of foreboding hung over me. I just had to be right, I had to be — but if I was, then why were the symptoms creeping back? Little did I know at this point that the cordless phones, smoke detectors, and electric clocks had EMFs and that if I pursued my search for the causes of what became a familiar cycle of ups and downs, I would find my answers.

Barrie, Ontario

As the summer came to an end, we watched each little family pack up and head for home. We too packed up, said our farewells, and headed for my second comfortable environment in the shape of a house that Lawrence had rented in Barrie. The house wasn't as idyllic as my parents' summerhouse, but it did have a big open space at the back. It was gas heated, situated on the edge of town near a farm, and there were no visible microwave relay dishes, no cell phone towers, and no power lines in sight except those that brought electricity to our street.

Initially we assumed we would stay in Barrie. Barrie had already proved itself to me and seemed less of a gamble than anywhere else. It was in Barrie that I had found my sanctuary, the one place I could always go to and know I would feel good. But after a week of Lawrence commuting to downtown Toronto, we realized that Barrie really didn't make any sense. Before we made any permanent change, we needed to be sure that the new location would satisfy all our needs. If I was going to continue to be sick or if Lawrence was going to become a single parent, he needed to be closer to home. So one of our main requirements was to enable Lawrence to continue as the breadwinner without a commute. Day after day we poured over the maps, initially of Ontario, but gradually further afield. We were, after all, transients already and there was nothing to keep us in Ontario. In comparing Newmarket with the places where I had been well — Barrie, Bridgton and Cambridge — we came up with a list of criterion of just what we were looking for: the conditions that would provide the best environment for recovery.

Essentially we were looking for an older, unrenovated house in a low density non-electric development on high, dry ground with a breeze, away from any microwave relays, cell phone towers, transformers, power plants, and power lines. Considering our financial state, our criterion seemed like a really tall order. But our search eventually led us to a hilltop in Calgary, Alberta, where we would have high ground, the possibility of escaping to the Rocky Mountains, and a city that used its natural resources of oil and gas for heating.

While Lawrence went off to Calgary to find a job and a house, the children and I remained in a rented house in Barrie for three months. Initially the three of us did well: the children soon brought home their back-to-school colds, but unlike the previous year in Newmarket where their colds had dragged on and they had both ended up on antibiotics, here their colds were what I expect colds to be. Their symptoms included a runny nose and a rise in temperature, but nothing that a couple of Tylenol couldn't handle. Within a few days they were fine and back at school.

What was really interesting though, was that during these colds, the children started coughing at night — those little hacking coughs that so often persist after colds. When I pulled their beds away from the walls, the coughing stopped. Repeatedly, instead of immediately tracking down the cough mixture when they began coughing, I would start by pulling their beds down and out from the wall — and within seconds their coughs were soothed and they fell into a deep restful sleep.

As in Bridgton, I also did well initially in Barrie. I continued to read; I had a whole new library to discover with a whole new section on health and well being where I discovered books like *Cross Currents* and *Healthy Home*. But after six weeks, my symptoms began to reappear — first the nightly seizures, then the tingling, weakening arm, and gradually problems with my balance. My comfortable environment gradually ceased to be comfortable and my excursions to my favorite spot on the lake increased, though at least now it was nearby. I could go over to the lake several times a day and get relief.

Calgary, Alberta

Within a week of leaving us, Lawrence had found a job with a company that was prepared to move us. He made an excellent choice of house — a bungalow on a sixty-foot lot overlooking a huge natural area. The overall ambient level of electricity from outside was very low and the unfinished basement gave us scope for moving wires if we needed to. It seemed that the conditions provided by this house were optimal for my recovery and I knew deep in my heart that if I were unable to find my answers in this environment, my options would be exhausted and I would have to resign myself to the care of conventional medicine. This was definitely going to be the end of the road for me.

We moved into our new house just before Christmas and as in Barrie and Bridgton, I was initially fine. But after about six weeks I began to worry that I had put my family through all these changes for nothing. My symptoms began to creep back — first the dizziness in the morning, then the tingling arm, and gradually the seizures. Our first year was very much characterized by ups and downs. For several days, even a week, I would feel good: my symptoms would be minimal, and I would feel that I was on the road back to recovery. But then suddenly my energy would drop and my symptoms would hit hard. Often I would feel despair: my symptoms seemed worse now than they had ever been. I would feel so disillusioned with the whole thing, that I would think, "Maybe it doesn't matter if my life is short if I have to live with these symptoms." Then after several days of being sick, I would begin to feel better again and the whole cycle would begin again.

Cycles of Symptoms

It took almost a whole year of these ups and downs before I connected these cycles with my electricity use. While I was well, I used electricity normally, building up quite a high ambient level inside the house: if the fluorescent light and the computer didn't bother me, I just left them on. When the symptoms began to reoccur, I wouldn't be well enough to use the computer, or to bake that batch of chocolate chip cookies for the children. With everything turned off, the ambient level of electricity in my house went down. Feeling better, I would again use electricity normally and raise the ambient level. So, in effect, while I was well I increased the demands on my body, thus making myself sick and while I was sick, I decreased the demands on my body thus making myself strong.

As I began to realize the mistake I was making, it became clear that I had to be much more diligent about which appliances I was leaving on when I was well. Of course, I couldn't work in the kitchen without light, which meant that the fluorescent light fixture recessed in the kitchen ceiling would have to be replaced by an incandescent light fixture as I didn't have any trouble with these. And weren't we surprised to find that the ceiling fixture harbored no less than six fluorescent light bulbs! Very soon the cycle of ups and downs changed: I would be up for the better part of a month and down for just a couple of days.

As I spent longer periods up and fewer down, I began to notice that I was very sensitive to appliances when they were in use. Even though the swing of the cycle was greatly diminished, there was a definite level of noise or disquiet when the computer, dishwasher, dryer, washing machine, or stereo was in use. I could even feel a difference when the computer was plugged in regardless of whether or not it was turned on. I began to insist that the children only play on the computer for an hour at a time because I didn't seem to be able to escape from the disquiet wherever I was in the house.

As my overall sensitivity to appliances heightened, I began eliminating them immediately, not giving them the opportunity to exert a cumulative effect on me which created fully-fledged symptoms. I gradually found connections to each of my symptoms. And with each connection that I made, I increased the amount of time that I spent up. I found that if I flicked the breakers on the electrical panel for the dryer, range, washer, dishwasher, garage door opener, computer, and microwave, I could achieve a tremendous level of calm in my head. I found that disconnecting the smoke and carbon monoxide detectors and unplugging electric clocks totally removed the tingling from my arm. Unplugging the stereo and disconnecting the ceiling fan removed my confusion, and changing my routine of playing computer games once the children were in bed to reading instead put a stop to my nightly seizures. In time my balance was restored, along with my thinking capacity, and my reaction to temperatures normalized.

Obviously, with so many electric circuits cut at the fuse box, the baseline of EMFs in my house was very low. As I became used to this standard, I would immediately begin to notice when anything was turned on. Fortunately this would not last for too long; the lengthy breaks from onslaught that I was able to give my body would soon enable me to have things turned on for several hours before they achieved a threatening level. But for a while I would notice the minute the children put batteries into their toys — and I'd take them out as soon as I saw that they were finished playing with the offending toy. Even battery clocks would create disquieting sensations. As time wore on, I would be able to cope with a heightened electromagnetic environment for several hours during the day. Not only could I count on baking and using the computer, but I was also able to go to the grocery store and to certain malls — as long as I didn't stay there all day and went home to my clean environment at the end of it. At night I would be careful to re-establish that level of calm by cutting the power to appliances at the electrical panel before I went to bed. Only the most necessary appliances and circuits received power during the night, namely the fridge, freezer, and bathroom light.

Of course with a family around me with its full set of comings and goings, maintaining an environment of minimized electricity took its toll.

The children had to get used to not sleeping with night-lights and not being able to turn on their bedroom lights during the night. They found my interference in their battery toys quite tedious, often reminding me that it was their toy. I even gave Christopher an electric clock for his birthday that played a drum rhythm as its alarm and had to replace it with a wind up clock because of the EMFs it emitted when the batteries were in. Fortunately, I found a really neat one with a transparent face that showed the clockwork working and the drum clock took up a position on his shelf as an ornament. The children couldn't, and still can't, charge their remote control battery packs while I'm in the house. Lawrence can't burn CDs and when my brother visits, he can only have power to his room over night if he agrees not to plug in his cell phone charger. More often than not my voice can be heard calling, "Supper's ready! Can you hit the range breaker?"

But for all the inconvenience of hitting electric breakers when appliances aren't in use, we are far less easily frustrated or annoyed than we were in any of our previous homes as a result of the lower level of ambient electricity.

After almost two years, I reached a state of health from which I could begin to resume some of my previous activities. I started swimming again. With everything I now knew about chlorine and swimming pools, I was very careful: I found a pool that used predominantly salt water and introduced myself to it slowly but found it fine. I began to take longer walks and, where at one time I had used the distance I could walk as a measure of improvement, I now had to stop myself because an hour of walking a day was enough. I tried downhill skiing though I prefer cross-country. I took the children skating and cycling along the Bow River. I even took up rollerblading. There had been many days when I thought I would never again have enough strength to live anything but a day-to-day existence. With each stride of my blades I cheered, "You were right, Angela, you were right."

As my life normalized and I regained my strength and energy, I became curious about the role that electricity had played in my downward spiral. Though initially the thought of electricity as my allergen had been mind boggling and filled with complexities, I had been able to find my way through the piles of information and establish an association between appliances and my symptoms. Though I was strong and well now, I wanted to know more. I wanted to know how something so safe could have robbed me of a year of my life. My mind still raced with questions. Was electricity affecting anyone else? What were they doing about it? What is that I could feel when the computer was plugged in but not turned on? Why did the carbon monoxide detector feel so different from the stereo? I wanted simple answers that made sense.

The more I looked at the research into EMFs in journals and books, the less they seemed to offer the kind of answers that explained what I wanted to know. They tended to look at the effect of specific frequencies on little animals or on specific appliances and power sources in relation to people. Research into cancer connections seemed to be a favorite but was far from answering my questions. I had managed to track down one website that sought to inform the public of the dangers of EMFs — the website of the Swedish Society for the Electrically Sensitive (FEB) which can be found at http://www.feb.se. Though there seemed to be few proactive measures on the FEB website, it did give me the reassurance that there were other people who were suffering as I had. Today sites such as this one are more prolific, offering an abundance of information on how to live with sick houses. Ultimately though it became clear that if I was going to get answers to my questions, I was going to have to go beyond the orthodox North American mindset toward electricity and its effect on people. Maybe if I continued my search for answers, I would be able to find a way of maintaining an environment in which I could remain healthy.

Part Two

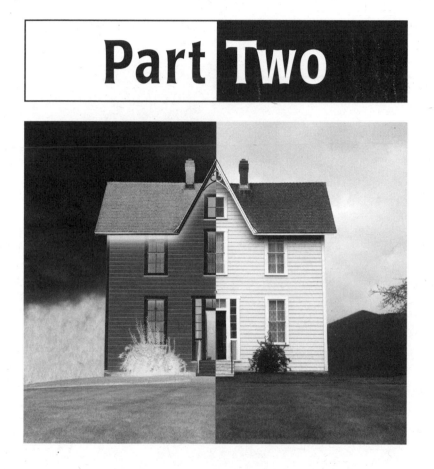

5

The Simple Steps

WHEN I WAS ILL, I WOULD HAVE GIVEN ALMOST ANYTHING for someone to hand me a list of things I could do that might help me to identify the cause of my symptoms and to get better. Despite my conviction that my symptoms had to be related to my immediate environment, there was no support and no concrete suggestion of how I could track down the cause. The information was out there, but it was all spread out in bits and pieces; putting it together into a usable format was daunting. Like so many of my fellow sufferers I was ready to look to expensive promises of cures and remedies such as detoxification hair analysis, pulse checking, and urine injections. But I discovered that there were things I could do that cost almost nothing except effort. From these, I have identified eight starting points which I have called the Simple Steps.

Figure 5.1 will give you an idea of the heavy burden we often, quite innocently, put on our bodies. We think of each of the burdens as being independent: we avoid one or other of them, depending on which we believe we are sensitive to. In order to really heal, I had to look at these burdens as a total load. The one that provoked a reaction was simply the last straw, as far as my body was concerned. I had to understand how the contributing factors interacted with each other and with my body.

The Simple Steps are based on creating the conditions in which the body's own healing mechanisms work best. If you look around you at the moment, you may find that several demands are being made on your body by chemicals and EMFs. You may be wearing a polyester sweat shirt, drinking a steaming cup of coffee while sitting in an overstuffed chair with your favorite music playing in the background. We take these things for granted: we don't even realize that

Mercury
from dental fillings,
vaccines, dyes
and glossy paper

Food Odors
during storage
and cooking

Food Additives
color,
preservatives,
emulsifiers, etc.

EMFs – Voluntary
*from sources within
our control such as:*
fans,
baby monitors,
dimmer switches,
televisions,
smoke/CO detectors
air purifiers, cell phones
microwave ovens,
security systems, etc.

EMFs – Involuntary
*from sources beyond
our control such as:*
satellites,
cell phone transmitters,
broadcast transmitters,
transformers,
powerlines, etc.

**Pesticides
&
Insecticides**

Chemicals
in cosmetics and
medicines

**Mold, Dust
Animal Dander**

Chemicals
in fabric and
plasticizers

Air Fresheners

Chemicals
in cleaners and polishes

Chemicals
in water

Chemicals
in air

Formaldehyde
in cosmetics, furnishings,

The Burdens Our Bodies Bear. **Credit**: *Angela Hobbs*

they are sources of chemicals and EMFs that place a burden on our bodies.

The chemicals around us enter our bodies not only from the food we eat but also from the air we breathe, the clothes we wear, the water we drink and bathe in, and the cosmetics and toiletries that come into contact with our skin. Once inside our bodies, they cause damage. Nature has put mechanisms in place to prevent this damage — for instance, it provides us with melatonin and a blood brain barrier. Melatonin protects us by neutralizing the free radicals that chemicals create in our bodies, and the blood brain barrier protects us by preventing chemicals from passing into the brain and spinal cord. Unfortunately, EMFs interfere with both of these protective mechanisms. They reduce the production of melatonin[1] which means there is less of this vital antioxidant available to deal with chemical damage, and they increase the permeability of the blood brain barrier[2] which allows chemicals to flow into the brain and spinal cord.

> Did you know that the hormone melatonin is the most potent antioxidant produced by the body? It helps to protect cells from the genetic damage that can lead to cancer and to neurological, cardiac, and reproductive damage.[3] The brain, hypothalamus, central nervous system, lymph system, immune system, heart, lungs, liver, kidneys, uterus, testes, and fetus all have melatonin receptors. Anything that affects the balance of this hormone affects organs throughout the body[4] — and EMFs affect the pineal gland's production of this hormone.[5]

By reducing EMFs, especially at night when melatonin production reaches its peak, and by minimizing the chemical burden that melatonin has to deal with, we can create an environment in which our body's own mechanisms can restore health.

The Simple Steps will show you how to create this optimal environment in your own home. Some of the steps may seem to deal with minute details: this is a reflection of the degree of detail I had to consider when attempting to create my own healing environment. You may discover that some of the steps are more informative than others, or that though you have reactions in certain places, they are not the symptoms you want help with. Depending on your reasons for pursuing the steps, you may want to adjust them to suit your own needs, or simply use them as a starting point for your own investigations. I recommend that you begin by completing Step 1, which includes a Daily Log designed to reveal connections between exposures and symptoms. As patterns become clear to you, you can go on to the worksheets that correspond to those patterns. For instance, if it becomes clear that skin exposure is at the root of your symptoms, go straight to Step 5 and Worksheet 8 which is designed to track your response to fabrics, cosmetics, and toiletries. Don't be afraid of making connections between your symptoms and your environment: anything in your environment can be provoking your symptoms and only your body can tell you what it is.

There are three basic goals that the steps aim to achieve: to identify and avoid the conditions that provoke our symptoms, thereby reducing the drain on our reserves; to remove the electromagnetic fields that hamper our hormones' ability to repair the damage that chemicals cause; and to create homes where our exposure to chemicals is minimal, giving our bodies a fighting chance to recover from daily exposure to chemicals over which we have no control.

To achieve these goals, the Simple Steps will show you how:

- to recognize the environments that provoke your symptoms through the use of comparison worksheets and a log;
- to find a place where you can sleep and how to create a sanctuary around it;
- to reduce your exposure to the chemicals in tap water;
- to use an elimination diet to isolate foods that burden your system and then reduce their chemical contribution;
- to limit the burden synthetic fabrics place on your system;
- to purify your air by eliminating or reducing sources of impurities — without creating additional burdens of electromagnetic fields generated by appliances;
- to decrease your exposure to electromagnetic fields by considering more than simply maintaining a "safe" distance;
- to balance your psychological, physical, and emotional needs.

Step 1:

Recognizing the Burdens Our Bodies Bear

The trademark of the symptoms of indoor pollution is their unpredictability, but you have probably realized that there are some places and times when your symptoms give you more difficulty. We tend to think that symptoms are related to indoor factors only if they occur indoors. However, our bodies are

Recognizing Sick House Symptoms

• **When conventional medicine tells us we're fine — but the symptoms persist.**

Though we need to pursue the resources of modern medicine, if discussions of our symptoms with several doctors leave us with conflicting or vague diagnoses, we should look at environmental factors.

• **When we know in the bottom of our hearts that something is wrong** — even though the blood tests come back telling us we're fine.

• **When other causes of our symptoms have been eliminated** — e.g., obvious stress, genetic predisposition, poor diet, external pollutants, etc.

• **When we have paid attention to the balance between our minds and bodies.** We know that the physical, spiritual, and emotional aspects of our lives are being nourished.

• **When our symptoms are inconsistent.** Do we always have them, or do they only appear in specific places? Do we have them when we go on holiday, when we go to our friends' houses, to the doctor's office — or do they only appear at work or at school? Do our rashes clear up when we go to the country? Do we only get migraines on weekends? Symptoms that tend to express themselves only in certain places are highly likely to be related to an overburdening of our bodies from elements in our personal environments.

initially weakened by conditions in the sick house, and thereafter our reactions can be induced wherever the conditions that provoke the symptoms occur.

In this first step you will see that if you know what you're looking for, many symptoms are readily predictable. For instance, if you suffer from psoriasis or eczema, you may have noticed that you didn't have it on holiday, that it gets a lot worse when you don't sleep, or a lot better when you don't go to work. By making comparisons, you may discover that your bed is close to the electrical panel and the symptoms abate when you move your bed. Though symptoms are often explained away as stress or diet related, in Step 1 you will be able to pursue other possible explanations.

There are three goals to this first step: to make sure, first of all, that you are working with symptoms connected to the indoor environment; secondly, to give you some early control over your symptoms by empowering you to recognize the combination of factors that brings them on; and thirdly, to put you in a position of strength from which to cope with the remaining steps.

By using the following worksheets, you can begin to isolate the places where you notice some variation in your symptoms, then go on to make more detailed comparisons that will help you to recognize the conditions which are most likely to provoke your symptoms. You can then make some immediate modifications to your environment, and use a daily log to help track the factors that affect your symptoms.

The Comparison Worksheet

To begin to identify the connections between your symptoms and your personal environment, fill in Worksheet 1. For each location in the first column, write in the appropriate column a brief description of any symptom that occurs in that location — always, sometimes, or never. In Column 1, add any additional locations in which you spend an appreciable amount of time, particularly if you suspect that it may relate to your symptoms. Columns 2, 3, and 4 are equally important: Columns 2 and 3 will help you to identify locations to avoid, and Column 4, those in which you can spend more of your time.

The "always" symptoms are those that you experience every time you are in a particular location. If you know that you will lie tossing and turning for hours every time you crawl into bed, then you would record "difficulty falling asleep" in Column 2 next to "bedroom" in Column 1. If you always get a headache when you wash the dishes, you would record "headache when washing dishes" beside "kitchen." If you always get anxious when you drive the car, you would record "anxiety when driving" in Column 2 next to "car" in Column 1.

The "sometimes" symptoms are often the most alarming. Knowing that something may jump out and get you but not knowing when or where can add an element of fear to already unpleasant symptoms. Your fear may already have made you avoid any number of situations. But if you don't know exactly what is causing your symptoms, the conditions that provoke them may still be lurking around the next corner. In order to provide the best conditions for healing, you need to analyze what contributes to the conditions that bring on your symptoms. You may be able to complete some of this analysis from afar, but you may also have to face your fear head on by returning to places that provoke your symptoms.

These "sometimes" symptoms also introduce the possibility that your symptoms are being provoked by a combination of conditions, or that they

Worksheet 1: *The Broad Comparisons Worksheet*

Instructions: For each location in Column 1, make a note of any symptoms you experience in the appropriate column—always, sometimes, or never.

Locations (1)	Always (2)	Sometimes (3)	Never (4)
Bedroom			
Family Room			
Office			
Kitchen			
Dining Room			
Bathroom			
Laundry			
Living Room			
Friend's house			
Mall			
Medical center			
Open area			
Restaurant			
Sports complex			
Classroom			
Car			

are delayed reactions. The detailed log on Worksheet 3 will help you to identify the specific conditions that provoke these symptoms.

The "never" column indicates the locations in which you should endeavor to spend as much time as possible. These are the places where your body has access to the low-burden environment that you will be working to create in your home. You may find clues to the conditions that provoke symptoms "sometimes" by comparing the details of the "never" locations with the details of the "always" locations.

The Detailed Comparison Worksheet

Worksheet 2 allows you to examine each of your symptoms in relation to the EMFs and the air quality in which they occur. Your goal is to identify what it is about your location that provokes your symptoms. The more detailed you can be about the sources of EMFs and the air quality around you, the more useful your information will be. The notes below may help you to identify possible factors in your environment that may be provoking your symptoms.

Column 2: External Power Sources

Are there any sources of power outdoors — power lines, cell phone transmitters, broadcasting transmitters, transformers, amateur radio masts, generators, etc. — within 100 feet of this location?

Column 3: Nearby Internal Power Sources

This refers to all the little and large appliances that you might find yourself next to — such as battery packs, stereos, computers, battery or electric clocks, smoke detectors, ranges, microwaves, convection ovens, televisions, dryers, washers, fluorescent lights, cell phone chargers, etc. — basically anything that uses electric power. Walls, ceilings, and floors may hide some of these appliances but not their effects! Think about what you would see if the wall, floors, and ceilings were transparent.

Column 4: Air Quality

Can you smell anything in particular — cleaning fluids, air fresheners, cooking smells, perfumes, molds, pets, etc.? Are there any obvious signs of dust, pet hair, mold, etc.? Are there any obvious places where they could be

Worksheet 2: *The Detailed Comparisons Worksheet*

Instructions: *For each location make a note in the adjacent columns regarding the conditions around you. Be as detailed as you can. Symptom being tracked:* _____

Locations (1)	Are you near external power sources? (2)	Are you near internal power sources? (3)	What do you notice about air quality? (4)	Other observations (5)
Bedroom				
Family Room				
Office				
Kitchen				
Dining Room				
Bathroom				
Laundry				
Living Room				
Friend's house				
Mall				
Medical center				
Open area				
Restaurant				
Sports complex				
Classroom				
Car				

hiding — overstuffed chairs, old mattresses, carpets, bookcases, old pianos, fridge cooling system, etc.?

Column 5: Other Observations

Does changing your position have any impact on your symptoms — for instance, sitting in a different chair, or moving your chair, bed, desk, or table a couple of feet in any direction? Other observations might include a change in symptoms at a particular time of day, after a good or bad night's sleep, significant weather changes, etc.

You will need one copy of Worksheet 2 for each of your symptoms, so if you have several symptoms, make several copies. Be sure to write in Column 1 any additional locations that you included in Worksheet 1. Write the name of the symptom that you are focusing on at the top of the worksheet, then go through the possible sources for that particular symptom.

Identifying Patterns

As you become aware of sources of burdens on your body, you may well notice patterns or combinations of conditions that provoke your reactions. For instance, that anxiety attack that takes hold the minute you walk through the mall doors may very well be provoked by the poor air quality and high EMFs that are so common in malls. You may find that there are some malls, or even just some mall entrances, where the conditions provoke your symptoms, and you may find others that don't.

Some obvious patterns may already have begun to emerge. You may notice that many of your answers are in a particular column: for instance, you may have realized that it's not stress that brings on your symptoms as you drive to work but rather the power lines above you or the leather upholstery in your car. You may have realized that watching television isn't your problem as much as the dust that swirls around you as you sit down in your over-stuffed chair.

Modifications You Can Implement Right Now

If your symptoms are particularly difficult during activities that require you to spend extended periods of time in the same spot, consider the details of your location and the air quality very carefully. There are several ways of modifying your location and changing the quality of the air around you.

Locations

Electromagnetic fields aren't fussy about walls, floors, or ceilings; most of them can pass right through. This makes it important to consider your location in relation to both the appliances that you can see and those that you can't. Is there a smoke detector or fluorescent light in the ceiling of the room below you, or is there one above you? Is there an appliance on the other side of the wall?

If you can't simply unplug or turn off power sources, both hidden and visible, then adjust your position to maximize your distance from them. Try other chairs, beds, desks, or tables to establish whether or not your reaction is related to your location.

Disk brakes, the steel wire reinforcing belts in radial tires, and the electric gadgetry in vehicles can create huge electromagnetic fields that can have a significant impact on symptoms. Try borrowing or renting a car with low levels — a manual Honda Civic or an automatic Nissan Quest — in order to track any changes in your symptoms.

Air Quality

Many synthetic fibers deliver their chemicals to our skin as our bodies heat them and cause them to offgas. This factor prevents the National Aeronautics and Space Administration (NASA) from using certain synthetic fibers on space shuttles! Substituting cotton sheets, sleepwear, and clothes, washing with unperfumed detergent, eliminating fabric softeners, and using unscented products can significantly impact the frequency of some symptoms.

Try using a foam or cotton mattress instead of a coil mattress. There is some suggestion that the coils of a spring mattress channel electromagnetic fields. If you use a foam mattress, be sure to use several layers of cotton sheets between it and you.

Chemicals you may encounter during extended activities include those that offgas heavily — from new televisions and computers during their first months, inks and chemicals involved in paper and printing, improperly or newly finished surfaces, leather, new furniture, and molds. In Step 6 you will learn how to reduce or eliminate these sources, but for now simply increase ventilation and get rid of anything with an obviously strong odor — scented candles, air fresheners, etc. Just ten minutes with all the windows open can completely change the air in a house.

Dust and mold that can provoke reactions can often be found in that favorite stuffed chair, the fluffy carpet, the dusty bookcase, forgotten corners, etc. Careful vacuuming and dusting with a damp cloth can eliminate much of the particulate matter. Use a damp cloth to clean moldy areas, because the vacuum cleaner may actually help distribute the spores.

You now need to avoid any environment that you have identified as provoking your symptoms. In these situations, your body is screaming, "This is too much for me, let's go!" By avoiding these environments, you stop using up your reserves which can instead be channeled towards healing. This avoidance is temporary — just until your body is strong enough to cope.

The Daily Log

The purpose of the log is similar to that of the Comparison Worksheets: it enables you to trace patterns between your symptoms and your environment. In the case of the log, however, it is important to repeat your observations on a daily basis. You may want to make sufficient copies of Worksheet 3 to enable you to keep the log for approximately six months.

At the end of each week, go over the daily entries to look for patterns. It may help to use a different set of colors to highlight each of your symptoms, another set to underline activities that cause difficulties, another set for appliances, etc. The colors may help you to see connections. Continue to do this every week for at least six months — and keep all your data.

In looking for patterns, bear in mind that symptoms can be delayed or may be provoked only by a combination of conditions. If it becomes clear that you are dealing with a symptom of this sort, try tracking everything in your log for three or four days, filling in each of the time frames even though you may not experience the symptoms at all times. For instance, even if your symptom doesn't appear until evening, fill in the morning and afternoon time frames. The headache that occurs in the evening may be related to the cleaning products you were using in the morning or to the clothes you were wearing when you went shopping in the afternoon.

The more aware you are of situations you need to avoid and the more burdens you can remove, the better the initial healing environment that you can create for your body. The notes below may help you to take full advantage of the Daily Log.

Symptoms

Record any symptoms or changes in symptoms that you experience during each time frame.

Activity and Location

What is your primary activity during the time the symptoms occur? What is your location during that time? Be as precise as you can: identify which corner of the couch, which area of the kitchen, etc.

Fabric

Could your reaction be related to chemical residues in fabric? Many of our easy-care synthetic fabrics release chemicals right onto our skin as our body heat warms them. Record the number of items you are wearing that are made from each fabric.

Cosmetics and Toiletries

In this column, record any cosmetics and toiletries you apply directly to your skin — for example, shampoo, conditioner, body lotion, soap, deodorant, perfume, etc. Use the specific product name so you can try alternatives later.

Appliances

Electromagnetic fields travel through walls, floors, and ceilings, so be sure to record any electrical appliances that are turned on, regardless of where they are in the house. Include them even if they seem small and insignificant, such as Light Emitting Diode (LED) clock displays, dimmer switches, fluorescent lights, battery packs, fans, microwave ovens, surge protectors, smoke detectors, carbon monoxide detectors, cell phone chargers, battery chargers, stereos, baby monitors, air purifiers, security systems, etc.

Air Quality

Is it particularly moist or dry? Are there any obvious odors? Odors can include anything from the mild fragrance of fabric softeners and toothpaste to the stronger odors of cleaners and car fumes.

Worksheet 3: *The Daily Log.*

Date:

Instructions: *As symptoms occur, record them in the appropriate time slot. Add a corresponding note in the adjacent columns to identify factors in your immediate environment.*

	Symptom	Activity & Location	Fabric	Cosmetic	Appliances	Air Quality	Food
M O R N I N G			Cotton: Wool: Polyester: Rayon: Nylon:	Shampoo: Body lotion: Conditioner: Deodorant: Soap:			Breakfast Snack
A F T E R N O O N			Cotton: Wool: Polyester: Rayon: Nylon:	Shampoo: Body lotion: Conditioner: Deodorant: Soap:			Lunch Snack
E V E N I N G			Cotton: Wool: Polyester: Rayon: Nylon:	Shampoo: Body lotion: Conditioner: Deodorant: Soap:			Dinner Snack
N I G H T			Cotton: Wool: Polyester: Rayon: Nylon:	Shampoo: Body lotion: Conditioner: Deodorant: Soap:			

Food

If you have never eaten basic foods, the prospect of having to fill in this table may well inspire you to begin. For the purposes of this log you just need to record food content — if you eat a potato you record "potato," but if you eat prepared French fries, you record "potato, canola oil, wheat flour, cornstarch, rice flour, salt, tapioca dextrin, spice, xanthan gum, color, dextrose, sodium phosphate" — whatever the package lists as ingredients.

With Step 1 complete, you may be amazed at the many different aspects of your environment that can combine to exert burdens on your body. We tend to think that everyone shares the same environment, but in reality, no two personal environments are identical. Even twins living in the same house will eat different quantities of nutrients, sleep in different concentrations of electromagnetic fields, and spend differing amounts of time on sustained activities. The burdens for each of them are determined by their individual location in terms of electromagnetic fields and by the load each bears in terms of the surrounding chemicals. The total of the burdens borne by each twin determines their individual health.

Step 2:

Finding A Good Place to Sleep

Sleep is a crucial element to healing and creating a healthy environment. It is during sleep that the hormones, primarily melatonin, that we rely on to cleanse our bodies, are produced in greatest quantity and are busiest. In order for these hormones to be most effective, we need to remove as many things as we can that stand in their way — we need to remove, or at least minimize, electromagnetic fields.

So often when people are sick, we hear them say something like, "The only place I can sleep is on the recliner in the living room." When we are sick, our bodies have a way of telling us that they need to sleep and where they would like to do so. When we don't feel well, we're inclined to give in to these intuitions, but the rest of the time we force ourselves to sleep in our beds. Our beds are positioned in our bedrooms with esthetics and practicality in mind, not electromagnetic fields and health.

"Yeah, right," I can just hear you saying. "Electromagnetic fields are everywhere, there's nothing we can do about them." The prospect of taking on electromagnetic fields may well seem overwhelming, but it is far easier than it seems. Figure 5.2 shows how electromagnetic fields can be divided up into layers: the natural layer that our bodies are equipped to handle, the unnatural layer beyond our control, and the unnatural layer within our control. In this step we are primarily concerned with reducing the layer within our control.

As electric and magnetic fields move through the air, they interact with each other and with obstacles in their path. While obstacles deter some electric fields, magnetic fields move through objects with ghostly ease — they penetrate walls, floors, and ceilings. When their paths cross, these waves of energy may cancel each other out, combine, or change direction. Ultimately this interaction creates areas where electromagnetic fields are more concentrated — pockets. (Step 7 talks about pockets in more detail)

The goal of Step 2 is to create optimal conditions for the production and functioning of hormones at night. This can be achieved by finding a place to sleep that is not located in a pocket of electromagnetic fields and by creating a sanctuary around your chosen sleeping place.

Selecting Electric Circuits

To take control over the electromagnetic fields in layers 5 and 6, you need first to get to know your electrical panel. If the circuits are not already labeled, label them. Have someone who is not suffering from sensitivities turn off the breakers one by one while you check to see which appliances are affected. Decide which circuits have to be left on through the night — the fridge, freezer, and a bathroom light would be an ideal minimum. The Germans have a device that does this automatically: their *spannunungs-freishalter* is attached to the electrical panel and minimizes the power to the house during the night.[6] The North American equivalent is the demand switch, which is attached to an individual circuit and eliminates all the power in that circuit until power is required.

When our homes are wired, we don't usually anticipate that we might need to minimize the power coming into our houses, with the result that circuits often don't divide neatly between rooms. This may mean that the bathroom light is on the same circuit as a bedroom or the television. An

Layers of Electromagnetic Fields

Natural	Constant	**Layer 1:** The earth's magnetic field, between 350 and 700 milligauss — the one the whales, fish, and birds use to navigate their way around the world.
	Fluctuating	**Layer 2:** The EMFs that accompany storms as they pass through our neighborhoods.
Unnatural and ***beyond*** our control	Constant	**Layer 3:** Satellites and communications networks, cell phone base stations, and television and radio broadcasting stations, etc.
	Fluctuating	**Layer 4:** Power lines, substations, transformers, etc. The EMFs fluctuate depending on usage.
Unnatural and ***within*** our control	Constant	**Layer 5:** Electrical appliances in our homes and offices that are on all the time — remote messaging systems, security systems, power packs, fans, smoke and carbon monoxide detectors, etc.
	Fluctuating	**Layer 6:** Electrical appliances in our homes that are on for short periods: washer, dryer, stove, stereo. The EMFs fluctuate depending on usage.

alternative to installing a demand switch is to unplug any appliances powered by these essential circuits for the night.

The seemingly innocent small appliances can be the most potent and penetrating of all — smoke and carbon monoxide detectors, dimmer switches, fans, baby monitors, and battery and electric clocks with motors that turn hands. Make sure that they are all unplugged. Deactivating smoke detectors may impact your house insurance and any claims you might have to make should your house burn down. Check your insurance company's position on disarming smoke detectors before you do so.

Before you settle down for the night, you need to establish a routine of flicking breakers and unplugging appliances. Sometimes it will seem arduous but it is very important because by reducing this heavy burden, you can begin to create an environment in which your body can regain its balance.

Worksheet 4 will help you to keep track of each item in your nightly routine. In the empty rows at the bottom of the first column, enter any additional locations or appliances that are specific to your living space. In the second column, record the number of the circuit in your electrical service panel that corresponds to the appliance or location in column 1. If the circuit is to be left off at night, check "off" in the appropriate column. If it is to be left on, check "on" and write down all of the appliances on that circuit that you want to unplug. Make enough copies of this checklist so that you can put one near the electric service panel, and one in whichever rooms have appliances that will need to be unplugged.

Avoiding Stimulants

Prepare for the night by eliminating any stimulants between six and eight hours before you plan to go to bed. Anything with caffeine in it — tea, coffee, Excedrin, soft drinks, chocolate (yes, even the chocolate chips in that chocolate chip cookie), plus any tobacco products. You may not think that they affect you, but it isn't uncommon for caffeine to take effect only several hours after it enters the body. Caffeine reduces melatonin production, as do some painkillers.

For at least an hour before you go to bed, avoid activities that involve the computer or close-range television screens — PlayStation, Nintendo, etc.

Changing Location

Now that you have prepared yourself for the night by minimizing your electromagnetic environment and eliminating any stimulants, you are ready to listen to what your body has to say about where it wants to sleep. This is particularly important if you have symptoms during the night, if it takes you unusually long to go to sleep, if you sleep fitfully, if you wake up feeling like you haven't slept, or if you wake up feeling awful and stabilize as the day goes on. For the next week, spend a night in several different locations until you find one where you sleep relatively well.

- **The Recliner** – If you already know that you get a great night's sleep when you curl up on the recliner, then try it for a couple of nights and see if it really is that great. If it is, but you find your position restricted, you might want to put your bed there.

- **Beds** – If you don't already have a spot in your mind, consider whether there is someone in your house who rarely gets colds or is

Worksheet 4: *Nightly Checklist of Electrical Circuits.*

Instructions: For each location make a note in the adjacent columns regarding the conditions around you. Be as detailed as you can. Symptom being tracked:

Appliance	Circuit	Off	On	Things to unplug that share this circuit
Washer				
Dryer				
Dishwasher				
Range				
Bedroom 1				
Bedroom 2				
Bedroom 3				
Bedroom 4				
Kitchen counters				
Kitchen counters				
Living room				
Dining room				
Office				
Den				
Bathroom 1				
Bathroom 2				
Garage				
Playroom				
Hall				

exceptionally healthy. Try sleeping in their bed for a couple of nights. You might also want to try sleeping in other beds in the house — and to try each one with your head at either end. There is some concern that the metal springs in mattresses may channel electromagnetic fields, so you may want to try both foam and cotton mattresses. Foam mattresses will need to be covered with several layers of cotton sheets to provide a barrier between you and the chemicals in the foam.

- **The Floor** – If you have no success with beds, then you may want to invest in a lightweight mattress that you can move easily. You need to move your mattress around the floor of your house by about a foot at a time. Think of your floor as if it were a grid of ten-inch squares. With each change, lie down and try it. If sleep just is not happening within a reasonable amount of time, move again. Keep your head at least two feet from any place where you know there is a powered circuit or a light in the ceiling of the room below you.

Children's night time coughing can be used to help you find good sleeping places. Moving children's beds a few inches from the wall can have a significant impact on their coughing. Start about a foot from the wall and then move the bed a couple of inches up, down, left, or right until the coughing stops. It can take quite a few moves, but once you find a good spot where they stop coughing, try it for a couple of nights. If it is consistently better than it was where the bed was originally positioned, arrange the other furniture around it.

Once you discover your sleeping place, you will be tempted to stop there and forget about the rest. Go ahead, indulge yourself: it's probably been a long time since you felt this good in the morning. But come back in a few days because there is still a lot you can do — you can still feel a whole lot better!

If, on the other hand, you have not discovered a sleeping place that has any impact on your sleep, don't lose heart. Make absolutely sure that your power consumption at night is minimal and move on to creating a sanctuary.

Creating a Sanctuary

The sanctuary has long been recognized among allergists as a method of reducing molds and particulate matter during sleep — allergens to which people have often tested positive. We use the sanctuary to reduce any unnecessary burdens on the body: the less our systems have to deal with externally, the more they can focus on healing internally. Continue to minimize electricity at night with the help of Worksheet 4, and use Worksheet 5 to track your reactions to your sanctuary.

Once you have managed to locate a sleeping place, you need to build up your sanctuary around it, adapting the basic elements to whatever extent your situation allows. If you have had no success in your search for a good sleeping place, it should actually be easier for you to create a sanctuary, using the following as guidelines.

Cleaning

Choose a room that is as far as possible from the electrical panel and as free of mold as you can make it. Remove everything from the room and cupboards and clean it thoroughly — wash the ceiling, floor, and walls with plain water to remove any traces of dust, and clean the windows and window frames. There are some low-odor, peroxide-based solutions at hardware stores that will prevent or at least delay the renewed growth of mold. But since our goal here is to minimize chemicals, you may just want to keep a close eye on obviously moldy areas and keep cleaning them.

When you are satisfied that you have removed every speck of dust, bring back the bed and make it up with cotton bedding. The bedding needs to be washed with an unperfumed detergent and triple rinsed. Nothing else should be brought into the room because of the possibility that dust can accumulate on it — you won't be keeping anything in the cupboard.

Initially, the sanctuary seems austere and sterile, but remember it is temporary — a tool that enables you to maximize your healing by minimizing the burdens on your body. Ventilate, dust with a damp cloth, and vacuum your sanctuary daily. Keep the door shut so that dust and mold from the rest of the house can't get in.

You may be tempted to bring in your air purifier, a heater, or a fan, but unfortunately these appliances will create electromagnetic fields that will hamper your progress. Once your sanctuary is free of dust and molds, you will have removed the impurities that an air purifier would normally be used to filter out. Utilizing the sanctuary during the warmest months will also eliminate the need for a separate source of heat. If at all possible, keep the power consumption in the whole house to an absolute minimum at night by unplugging appliances, removing batteries, and turning off breakers.

Carpets

Carpets are horrendous allergen traps and new carpets exude huge quantities of chemicals. If you can't remove them, then rinse older carpets thoroughly with plain water to remove as much dust as possible. For new carpets, make a barrier out of plastic tarpaulin that will prevent the chemicals from the carpet getting into your air. Cut the plastic into the dimensions of the room and hang it up outside for a week, exposing as much surface area as possible. Depending on your space restrictions (for instance, if you only have a small balcony), you may need to refold it several times, so that the whole surface has a chance to offgas into air that you will not be breathing. When you are satisfied that it no longer has an odor, spread it over the carpet, and tack it down before you replace the bed. The abundance of chemicals in new carpets and new floor boards presents far from ideal conditions for a sanctuary. If at all possible, sleep with the window open and ventilate frequently.

Use Worksheet 5 to keep track of the conditions your sanctuary is providing. For each day of the week, check the corresponding columns. Have you cleaned up those moldy areas? Are you monitoring your power at night? Have other appliances or furnishings crept in, and if so, what are they? Has there been any noticeable change in your symptoms? Make enough copies of this checklist to keep you going for a month. You may want to retain a blank one so that you can make more copies if you find that you want to continue to monitor conditions in your sanctuary.

Step 3:

Reducing the Chemical Burden – Water

The goals of this step are to heighten your awareness to the ease with which we, often unknowingly, consume chemicals, and to show you how to reduce these chemicals so that you can begin to give your body a healing environment.

In order to reduce your chemical burden, it is important for you to go through each aspect of your immediate environment, reducing the chemicals

Worksheet 5: *The Sanctuary Check List.*

Date:

Instructions: Each day of the week, keep track of any changes in the conditions of your sanctuary and any corresponding changes in your symptoms.

Did you...	Dust?	Vacuum?	Ventilate?	Clean mold?	Minimize power?	Add furnishings?	Add appliances?	Noticeable changes in your symptoms:
Monday								
Tuesday								
Wednesday								
Thursday								
Friday								
Saturday								
Sunday								

in the things that get into your body — beginning with the water that comes out of your tap.

Major Water Contaminants

Chlorine

Chlorine is added to tap water to kill bacteria, viruses, and some parasites. Despite these beneficial effects, it also reacts with organic matter to form trihalomethanes. Volatile trihalomethanes evaporate into the air, becoming a problem when we breathe them in when we take a shower or a bath, or use a swimming pool. Less volatile trihalomethanes remain in the water and enter our bodies when we drink it.

Aluminum

Alum is added to water as a coagulant to remove pathogenic microorganisms, organic compounds, and particulate matter. The amount that remains in tap water depends on several factors and, although most of the aluminum we consume passes straight through the body, the aluminum in water (which is in an unbound form) is absorbed. Aluminum affects memory, learning ability, and muscular control.[7]

Fluoride

Fluoride is associated with reduced tooth decay. According to Health Canada, approximately 38 percent of the Canadian population receives fluoridated drinking water.[8] While adults excrete up to 75 percent of the fluoride they ingest, children excrete much less because it is absorbed into their developing teeth and bones.[9]

Lead

Lead is a component of many plumbing systems and water that has been sitting for more than five hours may contain higher levels than water that has been run for a minute. Eating foods rich in calcium and iron allows less lead to be absorbed by the body.[10]

Of course chlorine, aluminum, fluoride, and lead are by no means the only impurities in tap water — countless other chemical residues are also present —

but this short list of familiar contaminants shows us how much we have to be aware of when we reach for our refreshing drink.

Boiling our water kills bacteria and makes the more volatile trihalomethanes, like chloroform, evaporate out. The overall impact of boiling on the water's content is minimal — it really does not take much out. Bottled water often seems like the perfect alternative but in Canada and the United States, tap water is tested more stringently than bottled water.

> Did you know that the consumption of bottled water in the United States has increased steadily over the last thirty years? In 1976 the average consumption was 5.7 liters, by 1986 that had risen to 17 liters, and in 1999 the average consumption was 35 liters.[11] Thirty-two percent of Canadians regularly use bottled water to avoid chemical contamination from their drinking water?[12]

Purifying Drinking Water

To reduce our chemical burden from water, we need to take out as many of the impurities as we can. Both reverse osmosis and distillation are recognized methods for removing impurities, and are usually combined with charcoal filtration to remove chlorine. Both systems have their strengths and weaknesses, but both provide relatively pure water. The equipment for both methods can be installed in homes, or the water can be purchased in blue bottles.

Today many grocery stores sell water purified by reverse osmosis, and it is worth noting that not all maintain their equipment to the same standard. Those who insist that the blue bottles be rinsed with bleach before they are filled are clearly missing the point, since adding bleach simply replaces the chlorine we are trying to get rid of. Rinsing the bottle with purified water should be enough. Specialty water stores may provide a more consistent product.

Purifying the Containers

The blue bottles used for purified water require soaking. During the first month, large amounts of chemicals leach into the water from the plastic. To avoid consuming these chemicals, soak blue bottles filled with regular tap water in a warm place. Empty them down the sink and refill them daily for the first month.

Glass bottles can also be used as containers for purified water. The main drawback is their sheer weight when full — but they require no soaking. Simple jug-type charcoal filters, which are inexpensive, also remove impurities, but to a lesser extent than reverse osmosis and distillation.

If you choose to maintain your own system for purifying water, take great care with the charcoal, which can become contaminated. Once it reaches a point of saturation, it not only allows impurities to pass, but may actually add impurities by re-releasing those it initially absorbed.

Purifying the Water We Bathe In

The chemicals in bathing water find their way into our bodies in two ways. Volatile chemicals evaporate from the hot water into the air we breathe and chemicals are absorbed through our skin. Our bodies can absorb more chlorine in a ten-minute shower than from drinking eight glasses of the same water.[13] To remove the chemicals from the water we bathe in, reverse osmosis units can be attached directly to the tap or shower. If the concern is primarily chlorine, a charcoal filtration system can be added to the tap or shower, or charcoal can be added to the resin base in water softeners. Charcoal filters tend to be less effective at removing impurities from hot water than from cold water.

Whichever method you choose, the goal is to remove as many impurities as you can from your water before you consume it or bathe in it. You may notice an immediate impact on your symptoms, or you may not notice any change at all. In either case, persevere: this is a relatively easy way of decreasing the total chemical load you are asking your body to work with.

Step 4:

Reducing the Chemical Burden – Food

Once you have reduced electromagnetic fields at night, created a sanctuary, and purified your water, your healing will have begun. Your hormones will have fewer new chemicals to deal with and there will be more hormones working to deal with those that do come in. To our hormones, it will be like that feeling we have during the Christmas holidays when everyone is home and the house is a constant mess. You reach a point where it seems that however much cleaning you do, you just can't seem to make an impact. For the hormones, removing the extra burdens would be a bit like the children going back to school, relatives going home, and husband going back to work. It doesn't take very long for our cleaning efforts to restore order.

There are still several significant sources of chemicals around you, and one of them is food. The chemicals, additives, and preservatives in food tend to be slow to encroach on our health. We try a new time-saving addition to our menu, everyone enjoys it, and before we know it, it has become a staple in our diet. Next time we do our shopping, another item sneaks into the cart. Soon Tater Tots replace potatoes, processed meats replace that lean slice of chicken, saucy prepared vegetables replace boiled carrots, and our salads, smothered in prepared salad dressings, come out of a bag impregnated with preservatives. We unknowingly consume significant quantities of chemicals, from food colorings, which are largely coal tar derivatives, to artificial flavorings, preservatives, and other additives.

Artificial flavor enhancers are designed to stimulate taste sensors in the same way that natural foods do, but because they are often incomplete replicas, they may lack the code that turns off the stimulation. The neuron is therefore left in its stimulated state until it disintegrates. This damage to our neurons can result in rapid mood swings, constant headaches, migraines, and Attention Deficit Disorder.[14]

Monosodium glutamate (MSG) is just one of many artificial flavor enhancers to watch for. MSG is found in yeast extract, autolyzed yeast, calcium caseinate, hydrolyzed protein, hydrolyzed oat flour, hydrolyzed plant protein, and often in natural beef flavorings, seasoning, or natural chicken flavoring.[15]

Preservatives include the nitrites that are added to smoked meats and hot-dogs to prevent botulism. The quantity added to hot-dogs is so high that eating more than one a month (or twelve in a year) elevates the risk of leukemia by 9.5 percent.[16] When heated, nitrites form highly carcinogenic nitrosamines. Additives often impact the texture of food. For instance, aluminum increases the creaminess of yogurt, nondairy creamers, and processed cheese, etc., but it also affects memory, learning ability, and muscular control.[17]

Children are particularly vulnerable to the additives in processed foods. They consume three times as much as adults for their weight[18] and are attracted by the bright colors, strong flavors, relentless advertising, and fancy packaging of processed foods. Their friends at school open their lunch boxes to chips, pudding cups, hot dogs, individually packaged cookies, sodas and jellies — how can a sandwich and juice ever compete? Their little bodies are forced to deal not only with pesticide and fumigant residues of unprocessed foods but also with synthetic additives that their bodies neither recognize nor know what to do with.

> **!** Did you know that a 1976 report by the US Food and Drug Administration estimated that 95–99 percent of children eat some foods containing dyes? By the time they are twelve, four million children will have consumed one pound of coal tar-based dyes and some as much as three pounds.[19]

Everything from brightly colored cereals, jelly, instant puddings, cans of soup to pizza pops and ready-made lasagna may be impregnated with chemicals after processing to restore the flavor and consistency that processing removes. Through these additives, the products achieve a level of consumer satisfaction with which basic meals can no longer compete.

Healthy eating has become synonymous with terms such as "low fat" and "sugar free." But our bodies are probably much better equipped to deal with natural fats and sugars than with the multitude of synthetic alternatives we use as "healthy" substitutes.

In Step 1, when you began recording all the food you ate, you may have been inspired to eat foods that are close to their natural state simply in order to make it easier to record the ingredients. The elimination diet will bring you back to those close-to-natural foods. You may have already used the elimination diet to find out if any foods are causing your symptoms: it is usually the first thing we try because it identifies common allergens. There is a lot of information about it and virtually all practitioners of alternative medicine advise their patients to start with it.

The goal of this step is to help you to recognize and eliminate chemicals in foods and to locate any foods that provoke obvious symptoms so you can avoid them. If you have already worked through the elimination diet and now avoid any foods that create problems for you, and if your diet already consists of foods that make a minimal contribution to your overall chemical exposure, you can move on to Step 5. If you are still unclear about the effect food may have on your symptoms, the next section, including Worksheets 6 and 7, will help you to identify possible sources of your difficulties in the foods you eat.

The Elimination Diet

The elimination diet exists in many forms, from the strictest variety, which begins with a fast, to the rotation diet, which leaves rest periods between foods groups, giving your system a break from digesting the same foods day in and day out. For our purposes, the elimination diet is a middle-of-the-road choice, because our purpose is not only to locate specific burdens, but to decrease the overall burden of chemicals that our bodies have to deal with.

If your regular diet consists primarily of processed foods, you first need to replace them with foods that are close to their natural state. That means that instead of frozen fries, you have to boil a potato. and instead of a Big Mac, you have to make your hamburger out of fresh meat. Any foods you eat that have more than one stage of processing should be replaced by foods with a single or no change from their natural state. A "one change" food is something you buy fresh in the produce section at the grocery store and change by baking, boiling, grilling, or microwaving yourself. The minute you add anything — such as salad dressing, bacon bits, seasonings (other than salt and pepper), or canned soups — these foods have gone through more than one change between being harvested and being consumed.

If eating foods this close to their natural state is a major adaptation for you, spend a couple of weeks getting used to them. Pay special attention to foods bursting with antioxidants — they will give your melatonin some much-needed support. These foods include broccoli, green peppers, black currants, avocados, watercress, sweet potatoes, hazelnuts, carrots, spinach, sprouts, and parsley.[20] If, on the other hand, you are quite comfortable with foods that are close to their natural state, get yourself started on the elimination diet with the help of Worksheets 6 and 7.

The Elimination Diet Planner

Begin by grouping the foods in your diet. Worksheet 6 will give you an idea which foods belong to which groups. If you prefer to create your own sequence, or already suspect that certain foods or groups of foods might be provoking your reactions, use Worksheet 7.

Next, abstain from anything in a single food group for the first four days of the week.

Gradually reintroduce these foods during the second half of the week — days five, six, and seven — paying close attention to your reactions. Take great care when reintroducing foods, especially if your symptoms have been noticeably different during their absence. Start with the smallest of portions and give your body several hours to respond. If you notice no change in your symptoms, then gradually increase the amount until you're back to your normal quantity. If, on the other hand, just a small amount provokes a reaction, stop reintroducing the food group.

Depending on the severity and nature of your reaction, you may want to pursue food allergies with a medical doctor. You might also want to try just a little of the food in its organic form, then take a complete break from that food group for several weeks and try again. For more information about food allergies, consult *Food Allergies: The Complete Guide to Understanding and Relieving Your Food Allergies*, by William Walsh, which is listed in the section on Recommended Reading.

Organic Foods

You may discover that a particular food — but not the whole food group — provokes your symptoms, and if that is the case, you might want to try the same food in its organic form. Testing suspect foods in their organic form will tell you if your reaction is to the food itself, or is caused by the many treatments it receives between being planted and being sold to you. Your reaction could be to the preservatives used to lengthen shelf life, to fumigants used in transportation and storage, to fertilizers, growth enhancers, and medications used to ensure maximum production, or to the gases used to artificially ripen produce.

In a study at Rutgers University, organic lettuce was found to contain five times more calcium than commercial lettuce and fifty times more iron. Organic tomatoes were found to contain five times more calcium than the commercial variety and two thousand times more iron.[21]

Restricting your diet to foods that are in season in your area may also help you to avoid some of the contaminants that result from storage and transportation over long distances. Make sure you scrub foods well or remove the skins. Simply rinsing does nothing to remove chemical residues since they are usually designed to be waterproof.

Do-It-Yourself Elimination Diet Planner

If you prefer to create your own table, use the blank one titled Worksheet 7. For example, you may already suspect that particular foods are affecting you

Worksheet 6: *The Elimination Diet Planner.*

Instructions: *For the first four days of each week, eliminate one food group from your diet. Over the last three days of the week, gradually reintroduce foods from this group. Record your reactions.*

Week	Abstain from:	Foods in this group:	Changes in reactions:
1	The beef group	Beef, veal, cheese yoghurt and other milk products	
2	The wheat group	pasta, crackers, snacks, lunch meats, sauces, cakes, cookies	
3	The pork group	Pork, lunch meats, bacon, ham, sausage	
4	The apple group	Apple, pear, quince, pectin, cider	
5	The poultry group	Chicken, turkey, eggs, duck	
6	The yeast group	Mushrooms, yeast, bread, wine, beer	
7	The citrus group	Oranges, lemons, grapefruit	
8			

adversely. To test this, create food groups that reflect those suspicions: for example, in Week 1, you might want to eliminate all nuts and food with nuts or nut oils. For each of the seven weeks, create a group of foods and enter it in the second column. In the third column, write the names of all the foods included in that group that you would normally eat. The sequence of elimination and reintroduction is the same: eliminate everything from one group for the first four days of the week, and gradually reintroduce those foods beginning on day five of the week. If you think you may want to keep trying different food groups, make several copies of Worksheet 7.

With the elimination diet complete, you will have achieved two things. You will have established which, if any, foods you should avoid because they provoke a reaction, and you will have significantly reduced the quantity of chemicals in your diet. With this lower consumption of chemicals, your body has fewer new chemicals to deal with and can concentrate on eliminating those that are already present.

Dangers in Preparing Foods

Aluminum

We unwittingly add the burden of aluminum during cooking. Its reputation for distributing heat evenly has led to its widespread use in saucepans and cooking equipment. Many of us are familiar with the method of cleaning silver using a sheet of aluminum foil and baking soda and adding heat in the form of boiling water. Unfortunately we may not realize that the chemical reaction that cleans our silver also occurs when we use aluminum foil to cover our food as it cooks. This same effect leaches toxins into the food as we apply heat before filling waiting tummies.

Plastics

The chemicals in plastics and Styrofoam containers leach into the food or liquid they hold, and the rate of leaching increases with heating. Though manufacturers claim that many plastic containers are safe for microwaving, remember that the claim is related to the containers' survival — not yours!

Worksheet 7: *The Do-It-Yourself Diet Planner.*

Instructions: *For each week, enter a group of foods that you want to discover your reaction to. For the first four days of each week, eliminate everything in one food group from your diet. over the last three days of the week, gradually reintroduce these foods. Record your reactions.*

Week	Abstain from:	Foods in this group:	Changes in reactions:
1			
2			
3			
4			
5			
6			
7			
8			

Stainless Steel

Stainless steel contains iron, nickel, and chromium. The safe intake range for chromium is 50–200 micrograms per day. One meal prepared with stainless steel gives about 45 micrograms of chromium.[22] The International Agency for Research on Cancer (IARC) recognizes chromium and nickel as known carcinogens.

Non-stick Coatings

Non-stick coatings are thought to be chemically inert, passing right through us harmlessly when they find their way from the pan into our bodies. Though the risk posed by these coatings becomes dangerous only if they are heated above 650°F (when they produce poisonous fumes),[23] most of us can probably think of preferable forms of roughage.

Step 5:

Reducing the Chemical Burden – Cosmetics & Fabrics

Your skin is designed to present a barrier to the environment and on the whole it does a great job. In Step 3 you discovered just how easily skin absorbs water and anything dissolved in it. Now you are going to find out about some of the other chemicals that our skin is exposed to through the clothes we wear and the cosmetics we use to keep it feeling soft and smelling fresh.

Regulations governing the chemicals in cosmetics vary considerably. American regulations require ingredients to be listed on cosmetics but do not require the chemicals to be tested before marketing. Canadian regulations are currently under review but at the time of writing only about a hundred chemicals are restricted; the names are not standardized and no list of contents is required. European regulations require cosmetics to carry a list of contents, chemical names are standardized, and over 450 ingredients are restricted.

The cosmetics industry is thought to be self-regulating: if a product hurts you, you won't buy it again. Unfortunately, in the case of cosmetics, by the time you realize that the product has hurt you, the damage is usually irreversible. We accept reassurances that the chemicals do not penetrate our skin because the molecules are too big, or that only huge quantities can have an impact, but sometimes it's what the chemicals prevent our bodies doing that causes the damage. For instance, studies on aluminum in antiperspirants tell us we cannot get cancer from antiperspirants. However, aluminum prevents our bodies from excreting toxins because it causes the cells in our armpits to swell, and it may be this retention of toxins that causes the problems.

Our misplaced trust in safety standards leaves us washing our hair with sodium lauryl sulfate, diethanolamine (DEA), and coal tar. Sodium lauryl sulfate is known to corrode hair follicles, impede hair growth, cause cell membranes to degenerate, and is thought to cause cataracts and blindness. DEA causes dermatitis and forms nitrosamines[24] — those same potent carcinogens that we watch for in smoked meats.

Recognizing the Chemicals in Cosmetics

For most of us the chemicals in cosmetics are as slow to encroach as the chemicals in food. We try a product that will untangle our child's hair so that we can brush it without the squeals. We lather on an antibacterial cream to limit the number of office colds we catch. "One bottle won't hurt," we think, "it wouldn't be on the market if it weren't safe." But gradually we get used to the soft skin, the relaxed hair brushing, and the chemicals become part and parcel of our daily lives. We add the next thing on the market — a product that will relax the wrinkles in our clothes, a new fabric softener — and so it goes. Unless we have an immediate reaction to the product we continue to use it.

In order to lift the burden on our bodies from chemicals penetrating our skin, we have to rethink our perception of luxury. When we step into our bath full of bubbly, warm, softened, perfumed water or the soothing hot tub, what do our bodies really think? Is our body's perception of luxury the same as the one advertised on the television or the bottle of bubble bath? Or is it cringing at the prospect of soaking in a concoction of chemicals used in engine degreasers and linked to symptoms that include a lack of concentration, hair loss, fatigue, cancer, etc. Maybe what our already overburdened systems need is a soak in pure water — a night off from the burden of all these chemicals.

Recognizing the Chemicals in Synthetic Fabrics

There are several synthetic fabrics: some, like acrylic, are a combination of wood pulp and chemicals while others, like polyester, are purely chemical. Synthetic fabrics are used in a variety of clothes and furnishings. Rayon lends itself to shirts, blouses, and skirts and acrylic is usually used to make knitted items. Polyester, on the other hand, is as versatile as cotton and the two are used almost interchangeably. Polyester's versatility and durability has made it the most common of the synthetic fabrics; we find it in an array of finishes, used in everything from underwear and pajamas to sheets and quilts, from carpets to furniture coverings.

Polyester's popularity has led us to accept it without question as to its safety. Most of us don't even know that it is chemically based and offgasses when heated. If this comes as news to you, try a simple test. Put a load of well-washed, triple-rinsed pure cotton in the dryer and take a sniff when it is dry and still hot. Now do the same for a load of polyester washed and rinsed the same way and take a sniff. That is the smell of the chemicals offgassing! This smell has spawned a whole industry producing an array of chemical fragrances designed to mask the smell.

Polyester is made from ethylene glycol, the same poisonous chemical that prevents automobile window cleaner from freezing. The cosmetics industry restricts its use in cosmetics intended for use over large areas of the body, but there is no similar restriction for clothing. The process of making polyester involves condensing ethylene glycol until it forms a strand. This strand is then woven into a fabric like any of the natural threads we make from cotton, silk, and wool. It looks much the same and depending on the processing, it feels much the same. We want to believe that in this solid form its chemical constituents are stable, just as we want to believe that the mercury in our amalgam fillings is stabilized by its combination with other metals.[25] It's not! If it were stable, it wouldn't smell when heated and NASA wouldn't have a problem using it in the confined area of space shuttles.

There's a good chance that if you take a look at all the clothes in your cupboard and the underwear in your drawer that most of them are made from synthetic fabrics, predominantly polyester. Don't worry: I'm not going to tell you to go out and buy all new cotton clothes and bedding — only to ask you to think about how you use them. Don't use any synthetic fabrics — and that includes nylon, polycotton, polyester, rayon, LYCRA, and acrylic — anywhere that they can be heated by the warmth of your body –which includes underwear, sleepwear, and bedding. Replace these with pure cotton.

Fabric Treatments for Odors

The biggest drawback of synthetic fabrics is the hazard that they add to our personal environments by virtue of their smell. Recognizing this disadvantage, a whole industry has grown up around them. A wide range of products have been added to the supermarket shelves that promise to hide, remove, or neutralize the smell. We can add perfumed softeners to our washer or our dryer, we can line our drawers with impregnated smelly papers, and we can plug in air fresheners, or spray them directly on to our furniture. What we are really doing is fighting the chemical smell with more chemicals.

> Did you know that ethylene glycol, which is used to make polyester, evaporates slowly at room temperature and readily when heated? The chemical from which ethylene glycol is made — ethylene oxide — has been linked to leukemia, stomach cancer, brain tumors, and possibly breast cancer, genetic damage, and birth defects in laboratory animals.[26]

With the exception of the common desire to hide the smell of sneaker feet, we seldom connect our use of perfumed products with the need to hide smells. In reality, however, that is what air fresheners are doing. Hard as it may be to believe, the contents of air fresheners are far more harmful to our air, than the unpleasant wafts from those sneaker feet. Many contain chemicals such as xylene that irritate the eyes and nose and cause coughing and hoarseness. At higher concentrations, xylene affects our reaction times, balance, and central nervous system.[27]

Fabric Softeners

The chemicals found in fabric softeners and dryer sheets are often carcinogens — such as benzyl acetate and limonene and camphor. Many cause central nervous system disorders, headaches, nausea, vomiting, dizziness, and a drop in blood pressure. Benzyl alcohol, ethyl acetate, linalool, alpha-terpineol, and many of these chemicals irritate the skin.[28] The need for chemical softening can be eliminated by using water softeners or by adding either one quarter of a cup of baking soda or one cup of vinegar to the final rinse.

The goal of Step 5 is to relieve your body of the burden that the chemicals in cosmetics and synthetic fabrics create. Here are some practical steps you can take to reduce that burden:

- Pay close attention to any cosmetics and synthetic fabrics that come into contact with your skin for periods long enough to allow them to be heated – even residues from washing powder count.
- Reduce the quantity of cosmetics and synthetic fabrics you use. You may want to replace your cosmetics and synthetic fabrics with natural alternatives. Keep in mind that not all natural products are safe, either.
- Replace polyester underwear, sleepwear, and bedding with well-washed, triple-rinsed cotton. Use an unperfumed laundry powder and don't add any fabric softeners.
- Wash new clothes before wearing them. New clothes are not only impregnated with sizing to make them hang nicely in the store, they also contain chemical residues from dyeing, finishing, and processing. Washing new clothes with a cup full of apple cider vinegar will break down many of the plasticizers that make a drop of water bead when it comes into contact with a dry item.
- When dry cleaning is unavoidable, hang the cleaned garments somewhere outside your living space to air out.

Tracking Your Response to Chemicals

Worksheet 8 will help keep you focused on reducing the chemical burden contributed by your fabrics and cosmetics. As you test each of the sources of skin exposure, use the chart to record your reaction (or lack of reaction), the alternative you found, and the date of use. Use the blank rows at the bottom of the worksheet to enter any additional items you normally use which expose your skin to chemicals. You may need several copies of the worksheet in order to continue testing for combinations of chemicals, so keep a blank one handy.

Testing Singles

To begin testing, give yourself two clear days where you wear nothing but well-washed and well-rinsed cotton — no deodorant, no shampoo, no polyester or rayon — just cotton. After these two clear days, expose your skin to one of the products that you want to test. Unless you have a reaction, continue the exposure for the amount of time you would normally use that product. For instance, if you've decided that two days without washing your hair is just beyond disgusting, wash your hair on this first testing day and then put the shampoo away. This is probably your normal exposure to shampoo, whereas your normal exposure to a polyester sweater might be sixteen hours.

If you have a reaction, stop testing and totally remove the item from your environment. Look for an alternative product, and test it, recording the date. For clothing, try similar items in natural fibers; for cosmetics and toiletries, consult *Home Safe Home: Protecting Yourself and Your Family from Everyday Toxics and Harmful Products*, by Deborah Lynn Dadd.

Whether or not you reacted to the item, leave one clear day between each test. On clear days, you can use the items that you have had no reaction to, but on test days, revert to pure cotton and no toiletries or cosmetics.

Continue with one day of testing and one day clear until you have completed your list of skin exposures.

Testing Doubles

Testing doubles is much the same as testing singles only now you have a baseline to begin working with combinations. Start with two clear days: these now include your cotton clothes and one of the items on your skin exposure list. This one item will be your "constant" until you have completed the list. That means that you can now wash your hair on the same day as you test, as long as your shampoo is the constant item on each day of testing until your list is complete.

Continue as you did with single testing, working with one skin exposure item for each test day and a clear day in between.

Once the list is exhausted and you have found alternatives for the problem items, begin testing again using another item on the skin exposure list as your constant.

Testing Triples

Testing Triples is just like testing doubles only now you choose two items from your skin exposure list as constants and test the remainder of the list. This will help with identifying combinations if you suspect that skin exposure is provoking your reactions but single and double testing has not turned up the culprit.

It's very easy to miss the skin contact source of chemical exposure as our cosmetics come creeping back: that new shower gel that you thought you'd just use occasionally, the new conditioner that left your hair so soft. As long as these treats remain occasional indulgences, they won't hamper your progress or the maintenance of a low chemical environment. Come back to the chart once a month and use it to keep yourself in check.

Step 6:

Reducing the Chemical Burden – Air

We spend an average of eighty to ninety percent of our time indoors, in air that is two to five times more polluted than outdoor air.[29] Many of our purchases offgas for several months, contributing a significant burden of chemicals to the air in our homes. The burden is greater in newer homes, where even the building materials make a contribution. Frequently, a lack of ventilation ensures that this chemical soup remains in the very place where we think we are safe from air pollution.

Recognizing the Source of Chemicals in the Air in Your Home

The goal of Step 6 is to help you recognize, reduce, and remove the sources of offgassing that create this heavy chemical exposure in your air. Here are some of the principal sources of this interior air pollution.

Formaldehyde

In that chemical soup, formaldehyde is probably the biggest offender. One in five people are sensitive to formaldehyde and it is often a factor in the onset of sensitivity to chemicals.[30] Formaldehyde is a neurotoxin, but it is also a useful chemical found in disinfectants and preservatives, glues, pressed board, plastic, cosmetics, inks, vaccines, wood floors, new carpets, linoleum glue, new particleboard, cabinets, etc. The International Agency for Research on Cancer (IARC) classifies formaldehyde as a probable human carcinogen and the EPA refers to it as a hazardous substance and hazardous waste.

Most of us remember the fuss about removing urea formaldehyde foam insulation (UFFI) from our homes. Today in many states and provinces,

Worksheet 8: *Tracking Responses to Fabrics and Cosmetics.*

Instructions: *Once all products that smell have been placed in sealed containers or removed from your living space, reintroduce one product at a time. Note any symptoms, then return the product to its safe storage space. If you have a reaction, substitute an alternative product and note your reaction to that.*

Skin Exposure (1)	Reaction (2)	Alternative Product (3)	Change in Reaction (4)
Polyester			
Nylon			
Rayon			
Acrylic			
Polycotton			
LYCRA			
Bubble bath			
Shampoo			
Conditioner			
Soap			
Body lotion			
Deodorant			
Anti-perspirant			
Washing powder			
Dry cleaning			
New clothes			

when you buy a house, the owners are obliged to divulge if there is any UFFI in the walls, and books on buying a house include information on checking for telltale signs of the presence of UFFI. In this context, formaldehyde has had its day in the sun. Much less publicized is the presence of formaldehyde in building materials and the high levels of it that can often be found in new buildings, especially those lacking adequate ventilation.

Epoxy – Not Just Glue!

Epoxy is most familiar to us as the glue used to adhere our linoleum and wood flooring. Less familiar, but more dangerous, is its use in making the circuit boards in computers. Often computers are placed next to beds; some bunk beds are even designed to accommodate them directly under the top bunk.

The offgassing from computers drops quickly during the first year, but continues for years. Aware of the effect these toxins have on their employees' judgment, some companies install special ventilation systems, while others leave new computers to burn off for a couple of weeks before they are used. All over the world, women who have suffered miscarriages and spontaneous abortions wonder if their computers might have played a role.[31] It is thought that the poisons offgassed by computers and televisions probably have a greater impact on pregnancies than the EMFs that they create. But bearing in mind that EMFs amplify their effect, could it be that the combination of EMFs and chemicals is at work here? Could it be that our proximity to computers adds its own little boost to the process?

The significant contribution to air pollution from chemicals released by computers is given little recognition in schools. Our children are educated in sealed classrooms lined with "ready-to-use" computers — yet we attribute their headaches and nausea to everything but the air they breathe.

Cleaning Fluids

Most of us are far more particular about checking our information sources at work than at home. Often we don't really even think of our cleaning fluids as chemicals — popping a pellet into the toilet will keep it clean for weeks, a spray of shower cleaner will keep our showers sparkling, treating our mattresses and carpets with Scotchgard will stop stains and keep them looking clean and fresh.

As we walk through our homes, we relish the thick pile of the carpet, the comforters on the beds, and the cupboards overflowing with clothes. We cast a cursory glance at the toys the children didn't pick up and we curl up in the overstuffed armchair, reveling in the luxury that surrounds us. Taking another look, from the perspective of our new awareness of the chemicals that our "luxuries" offgas into the air we breathe, leaves us with a completely different picture. We begin to notice the foam padding that makes the carpet so bouncy, the synthetic fibers and

Did you know that 3M Corporation began phasing out its $3 hundred million fluoro-chemical business that makes the chemical in Scotchgard because the perfluoro-ocanyl sulfonate compound was found to be more persistent than PCB and DDT and has spread around the world accumulating in animals in remote areas?[32]

chemical treatments that make the carpet so soft and enticing, the foam padding and polyester stuffing that makes that overstuffed chair so welcoming.

With so many chemicals pouring into our air, it is hardly surprising that we reach for air fresheners. Relying on synthetic chemicals and electric gadgets to improve our air quality may do the complete opposite. Air purifiers provide another source of EMFs and air fresheners often include xylene, a chemical that irritates the eyes and nose, causes coughing, slows reaction times, and affects our central nervous system and balance.[33]

Mold

Mold can be a significant source of toxins, especially in the cool evening air and damp places. As the first snow and freezing temperatures arrive, molds tend to be less troublesome. Sources of airborne molds include:

- damp poorly ventilated rooms and basements that flood;
- hampers containing unwashed or damp clothing;
- storage areas, closets, and drawers;
- old upholstered furniture, old wallpaper, and carpeting;
- old newspapers and books;
- leaky roofs, windowsills, and showers;
- humidifiers and air-conditioning systems;
- decaying leaves, grass, and plants.

Food Odors

Many foods add an extra burden to our systems by adding odors to our air. Spices are a pretty obvious one (and should be kept in sealed containers), but brown sugar, herbal tea, fresh bread, etc. can also be significant. Work your way through your food cupboard and put anything that has an odor into a sealed glass container.

The smells from cooking and baking can be quite strong, penetrating, and lingering. Even something as basic as brewing a pot of coffee can add a significant burden to an already weak body. In the open plan house, these odors can be very difficult to control. Ventilate as much as you can and try to prevent them from spreading through the house if at all possible.

Eliminating and Reducing Sources of Indoor Air Pollution

If we approach air purification with the intention of removing the sources of contaminants, we remove the need for artificial forms of air purification and for air fresheners. We can leave things to offgas in a separate air space — essentially, an area that cannot contaminate the air inside our living space. Here are some of the ways you can minimize indoor air pollution:

- **Ventilate**. Opening all the windows for fifteen minutes changes the air in the whole house. Discard air fresheners and ban any smoking indoors.

- **Store household chemicals in a separate airspace**. Try using the garage, balcony, or shed. Such products include cleaning fluids and powders, such as laundry soap and detergents. (You only need to walk down the cleaning aisle at the grocery store to know that cleaning products leach their chemicals through plastic containers.) For convenience, store a small amount of dishwasher and dish detergent in small sealed glass containers in the kitchen. Paints, paint thinners, and any chemically based decorating accessories should always be stored well away from living space.

- **Give new furnishings time to offgas in a separate air space**. This can take several months. Buying floor models that have already had a chance to offgas in the showroom is worth serious consideration. Some carpet stores will air out carpets before fitting.

• **Seal surfaces that exude formaldehyde.** Any particleboard surfaces that are open to the air can be sealed with self-adhesive aluminum tape. This tape gives a good seal without exposing you to the chemicals during the offgassing period of liquid sealants. Some places that may not seem obvious include shelf edges, the underside of counter tops, and the underside of laminated furniture.

• **Store foods and spices that have an odor away from your living space.** Foods that need to be accessible can be stored in sealed glass or metal containers.

• **Store necessary cosmetics and personal hygiene products in sealed glass or metal containers.** This includes such everyday products as toothpaste and shampoo. Any such products that do not need to be constantly accessible should be stored in a separate air space.

• **Seal off moldy areas so that they have no access to your air.** Pay special attention to holes where pipes come up through the floor. Plants can be a source of mold and chemicals; find them a new home until you are better.

• **Keep any newspapers in the separate air space.**

• **Remove flea collars from the living space.** Like many air fresheners, these contain xylene; avoid using them in the house if you can.

• **Seal off any home office areas.** Printers, copiers, and fax machines are a significant source of chemicals.

Once all products that smell have been placed in sealed containers or removed from your living space, you can use Worksheet 9 to help track your responses to the chemicals in your air. Reintroduce one product at a time and make a note of any reaction you have; then return the product to its safe storage place. If you do have a negative reaction, try using an alternative product and note your reaction to that. Suggestions for alternatives for almost every home product can be found in *Better Basics for the Home: A Complete Guide for Creating a Healthy Indoor Environment*, by Lynn Marie Bower. (See Recommended Reading for further information on this and other books on this subject.)

It is easy to get quite relaxed about keeping the sources of chemicals out of your air. As you begin to feel better, the curry powder gets left out, the shampoo bottle doesn't make it back into its container, and you don't have time to ventilate. Use the Worksheet to keep yourself in check.

Pay particular attention to these sources in winter. Sealed houses during winter can increase our chemical load. The chemicals from our carpets, furnishings, cleaning products, cosmetics, and foods accumulate in our air — but we don't want to open windows and let out our heat. However, ventilation is just as important during winter, especially when we consider all the extra chemical sources that we bring in — Christmas trees with their pesticides, chemical pine scents, baking fumes, gifts made of new plastic, unwashed clothing impregnated with sizing, glossy wrapping paper impregnated with mercury inks, etc.

Worksheet 9 is intended to help you isolate products that cause a reaction, much the way the Elimination Diet helped you to identify allergies to foods. Make a note of any symptoms you have when handling a particular product; try using alternative products until you find one that doesn't provoke a reaction. Does the symptom disappear when you take these products out of your air space? If so, either eliminate the product or store it away from your living space. Use the empty rows at the bottom of the worksheet to add any other sources of chemicals in your living space.

Step 7:

Reducing the Electromagnetic Fields Around Us

Now that you have removed the chemical burden by working through your water, food, fabric, and air, it is time to consider the many sources of electromagnetic fields (EMFs) that you are exposed to during the day. In Step 2 you learned how to switch off your circuit breakers at night and

Worksheet 9: *Tracking Responses to Chemicals in the Air.*

Instructions: *Once all products that smell have been placed in sealed containers or removed from your living space, reintroduce one product at a time. Note any symptoms, then return the product to its safe storage space. If you have a reaction, substitute an alternative product and note your reaction to that.*

Product	Reaction	Alternative Product	Reactions to Alternative
Washing powder			
Dish detergents			
Cleaning fluids			
Fabric softener			
Window cleaner			
Air freshener			
Plants			
New furniture			
Craft supplies			
Newspapers			
New plastic toys			
New shoes			
Dry cleaning			

unplug appliances on powered circuits. The total impracticality of turning off all the breakers during the day means that you need to know something about the EMFs your appliances create. Only by knowing about these fields can you be sure you don't expose your body for extensive periods to EMFs that can make you sick.

Because EMFs affect the production of melatonin and its ability to clean the body, they amplify the impact that chemicals have on us. Toxins that should be eliminated from our bodies remain and begin interfering with the body's normal functioning. In order to create the optimal environment for our hormones to efficiently eliminate chemicals from our bodies, we have to remove the EMFs that hamper their progress. Researchers have established that EMFs affect our hormones, and have connected EMFs with behavioral changes, including anxiety, stress, disorientation, cancers, tumors, and disorders of the central nervous, immune, metabolic, cardiovascular, respiratory, and reproductive systems. It is suspected that EMFs may also play a role in neonatal death, spontaneous abortion, sterility, cancer, and genetic damage.[34]

How Much Is Too Much?

There is a great deal of debate about the health effects of EMFs, and a huge difference between what the Eastern and Western world consider to be safe exposures. Traditionally, the Western world's safety standards have been based on a belief that EMFs must cause heating to have any impact on health. The safety standards of the Eastern world reflect their belief that creating heat is not a prerequisite. To us, this means that depending on where you are in the world when you ask if your EMF exposure in your kitchen is safe, the answer will vary: in Russia you will be told "no" and in North America you will be told "yes," and in any country in between the response will reflect the influence of Russia or America.

The general rule of thumb when we seek advice about electricity is that we can minimize our exposure to appliances by maintaining a distance of two to three feet. This "safe" distance is tied to the idea that our exposure is limited because we don't spend the whole day, every day, in the kitchen with all our appliances on. The Specific Absorption Rate (SAR) is used as a guideline for people whose work requires them to spend extensive periods in high exposure environments — electricians who work on power lines, for instance.

"Safety" Standards for Some Common Household Appliances

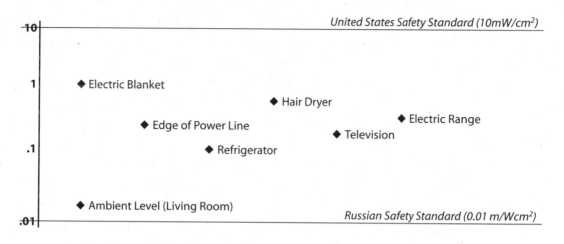

The Russian and American military conducted the bulk of the research into EMFs that led to the safety standards in effect today. While Russian research led to a standard of 0.01 milliwatts per square centimeter, American research led to 10 milliwatts per square centimeter — 1,000 times higher! — where it has remained since the 1950s, despite warnings that this standard is too high. [35] As this figure shows, the EMFs produced by our appliances exceed the the Russian standard while remaining within the US safety standards.

At first sight, the argument for a "safe" distance from our everyday power sources would seem to offer us protection from the doses of EMFs known to have health effects, but this is contradicted when we realize that we use frequencies around 60 hertz to navigate and to communicate with distant ships and deeply submerged submarines. Stepping back three feet hardly seems worth the effort.

Yet the proximity of residences, nursing homes, schools, and daycare centers to power lines, cell phone towers, television transmitters, etc., attests to our belief that nothing happens beyond the "safe" distance. But in an age where devices that emit EMFs are proliferating at a rate that would put rabbits to shame, the environment for which the safety standards were created has changed.

What Does Today's Environment Look Like?

Today's home environment looks very different than it did in the 1950s and 1960s when only the fridge emitted EMFs intermittently through the night.

> **!** Did you know that it is very possible that our increased consumption of the whole EMF spectrum may be related to the concurrent rise of allergies, asthma, cancers, autism, Parkinson's, multiple sclerosis, Alzheimers, Sudden Infant Death Syndrome, learning disabilities, depression, nervous disorders, etc.?[36]

Today's home is full of transformers, power packs, smoke detectors, security systems, carbon monoxide detectors, dimmer switches, battery clocks — the list seems endless. Each of these devices is a source of EMFs, nicely spread around our homes guaranteeing that they will interact with us and with each other from every direction. Figure 5.4 gives you an idea of the strength of the EMFs created by some of the appliances in our homes.

When EMF exposures are recreated in the lab, researchers tend to work with measurable, manageable, compartmentalized chunks of the electromagnetic spectrum, recreating them from just one source. These re-creations bear little resemblance to the reality of our exposure. They resemble the EMF environment on Pluto rather than on Earth, but these are the exposures on which our safety standards are based. The EMFs that surround us come from everywhere — inside, outside, left and right — they are multidirectional and multisourced. These fields interact with each other and with obstacles, setting up something much more akin to spiders' webs in an abandoned barn than to the nice little array of a single, lonely fridge on Pluto.

Understanding EMFs – An Analogy

Pebbles

To get an idea of the interacting EMFs around you, imagine for a moment that you are standing beside a calm lake. You throw a pebble, and watch as ripples radiate out from the place where the pebble hit the surface of the lake. Unless you throw in another pebble, the water soon becomes calm. Now imagine throwing in a handful of pebbles. The ripples radiate out from each pebble until they meet. When they meet, they interact and if anything obstructs their path, they interact with that, too. This interaction causes a change to the ripple — we might see a little crest, a change in direction, calm

Some Home Appliances That Generate EMFs

Low magnetic fields measuring less than 30 milligauss at six inches are created by:

Baby monitors	Electric ovens	Irons
Battery chargers	Electric ranges	Stereos
Clothes dryers	Fax machines	Toasters
Coffee makers	Food processors	VDT's
Crock pots	Fridges	

Medium magnetic fields measuring between 40–100 milligauss at six inches are created by:

Blenders	Electric clocks	Mixers
Copy machines	Garbage disposals	Sewing machines

High magnetic fields measuring between 110–200 milligauss at six inches are created by:

Air cleaners	Fluorescent lights	Pencil sharpeners
Dishwashers	Hair dryers	Smoke detectors
Electric drills	Microwave	Washing machines
Electric razors	Ovens	

Very high magnetic fields measuring above 200 milligauss at six inches are created by:

Can openers	Carbon monoxide detectors	Vacuum cleaners

patches and rough patches. This interaction continues for as long as we continue to throw in pebbles.

The appliances in our homes are very much like the pebbles. Around the appliance the electromagnetic field is consistent, but beyond a certain point, these waves of energy become inconsistent as they begin interacting with other waves and obstacles. The more appliances that emit EMFs, the more pebbles are contributing their ripples to the immediate environment — making more ripples that interact with each other. As long as we provide power to these appliances, the ripples and their interactions continue.

The analogy to pebbles and ripples on the water's surface gives us an idea of the movement of EMFs on a single plane. EMFs, however, radiate in all directions — from the front, back, top, bottom, and sides of appliances. To get an idea of what that would look like, we have to imagine moving that single cross section of the lake's surface through every degree and on every plane. If we now consider these fields in relation to obstacles and to the other layers of electromagnetic fields, a picture develops of an abandoned barn where the spiders' webs have taken over. Some areas have far greater concentrations than others, depending on the conditions they provide. If we could see these concentrations as pockets of EMFs, we would think twice about curling up with a good book or expecting a restful night's sleep amongst them. Because we can't see these pockets of concentrated energy, we force our bodies to remain in them and either take something to ensure a good night's sleep or accept the symptoms that result. We would do better to pay attention to our body's reaction to the EMFs and move when we're uncomfortable.

Our whole perception of EMFs is that they somehow become non-existent beyond two to three feet. When we acknowledge their presence beyond this "safe" distance, we can begin to understand the reality of our exposure at home and to discover how we can use this information to create healthier homes. We begin to see how turning on the stove might affect the concentration of EMFs around our favorite chair in the family room, or how turning on the stereo might affect the concentration around the desk in the bedroom. Suddenly connections between the electricity around us and our symptoms become obvious. Maybe we don't sleep well in our beds since we moved them because the move put our heads into a concentrated pocket of EMFs; maybe that spontaneous remission we're experiencing has less to do with spontaneity than with a recent re-arrangement of our appliances.

Since moving, adding, or removing an appliance changes the location of EMF concentrations, any symptoms related to them will also change. As we change the angle of the approach, we change the interaction of EMFs — and thus the location and the size of the pocket.

Reducing Exposure to EMFs in Our Homes

The goal of this step is to provide the optimal conditions for the production of the melatonin by decreasing our exposure to the EMFs that reduce its efficiency. In order to achieve this we have to consider both our proximity to anything that uses power during periods of extended activity and our location in relation to the pockets that result from the interaction of the energy being given off by our appliances.

Find the Safe Spots

When you position yourself for an extended period, consider both the sources of EMFs that are visible and those on the other side of the wall, ceiling, or floor. Only some EMFs are deterred by obstacles. In Figure 5.5, X marks the places where you should not spend extended periods. When choosing where to place a bed, consider the position of any ceiling-mounted fluorescent lighting and smoke detectors — and remember, the ceiling of one room is the floor of another.

Did you know that the first cases of multiple sclerosis in the remote Faeroe Islands appeared three years after the arrival of British troops and occurred in areas around their communications and radar stations?[37]

Check the Wiring

Have an electrician relocate any wires that run under beds or chairs where you spend extended periods. Bear in mind that wires carrying unused electricity behave like antennae. Electricity that comes into our homes moves

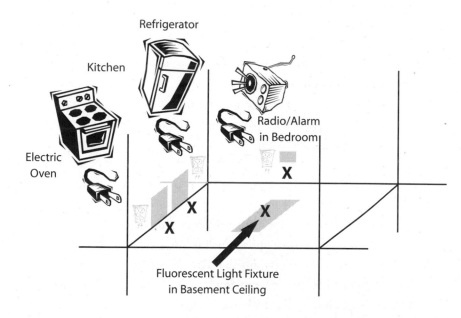

Hidden Dangers in an Empty Room. In this central room, X marks the spot in which you should avoid remaining for extended periods.

to an appliance where it is used to create, light, heat, sound, etc. If it arrives and is not needed, it heads back down the wire. In traveling to and fro, up and down the wire, the electricity in the wires behaves just like the electricity in antennae. The only difference between the wires in your house and the wires designed to transmit signals is the length of the wire. The proportion of the wire to the wavelength determines an antenna's efficiency.

Have the electrician check for faulty wiring or grounding to the plumbing.

Reduce the Pockets

Thinking back to that handful of pebbles, we realize that the only way to restore the water's calm is to stop throwing pebbles. By unplugging appliances we can limit the number of pebbles emitting EMFs and the areas of concentration they create. Pay particular attention to power packs, battery chargers, analog clocks (including battery operated ones), and anything with a Light Emitting Diode display (LED). Some of our smallest appliances emit larger than life fields.

Avoid the Pockets

If you notice that there are places in your house where your symptoms seem more intense, you may well have discovered a pocket. Avoid spending extensive periods there. The longer we spend in close proximity to EMF sources and the more time we spend in areas of high concentration, the greater their toll on our health.

You may find that in the early stages you recover more quickly if you maintain your nighttime EMF levels throughout the day, turning on circuits at the electrical panel only when you need them. Alternatively, you may discover that it is more convenient to limit the number of appliances that are plugged in. The extended periods that you spend in calm areas, where EMFs don't concentrate, will decrease your overall dose of EMFs. In these areas your hormones won't be disturbed; they can be produced at capacity and work efficiently. In these optimum conditions, especially at night, your body can gain ground on the toxins that have built up in your body.

Use Worksheet 10 to keep track of any reactions you may have to the electrical equipment in your home. Figure 5.6 gives a list of equipment that is often plugged in for extended periods. Once you have unplugged as many of these devices as possible, those that remain become part of your baseline — the minimum possible use of appliances that generate EMFs. Your baseline will probably include the fridge, freezer, and hot water tank, but — depending on the amount of cooperation you can elicit from the other people in your house — it may also have to include such things as the coffee maker, the computer, or sound system. It must not include surge protectors, fluorescent lights, or battery chargers. As deactivating smoke detectors may affect your house insurance and any claims you might have to make regarding fire damage, check with your insurance agent before disarming smoke detectors. You will need to keep this baseline constant during the day for the next two weeks.

Across the top of Worksheet 10, write the names of the appliances you unplugged — that is, everything that isn't part of the baseline but which is in use for extended periods of time. Use the list in Figure 5.6 to help jog your memory of some of the less obvious electrical equipment in your home. Then make enough copies to keep a daily record for two weeks. If your home includes a great many electrical appliances, you may need more than one sheet per day to enter all the items you are tracking. For each day of the two week period, record your use of each appliance, entering the time you turned it on, the time you turned it off, and any reactions, including the time they appeared and how long they lasted.

As you review your daily entries, look for patterns between your symptoms and the appliances in use. If it becomes clear that a particular device is provoking a reaction, you may have to stop using it for a while. If you identify problems arising from working with equipment that is indispensable — things that you use to earn a living, for instance — you may want to try these alternatives:

- Use the appliance in another location. The concentration of EMFs around the appliance may be affecting you more than the EMFs produced by the appliance itself.
- Use a similar appliance. Not all appliances are created equal: where one computer may send you running for cover, another may have no effect on you at all.
- Distribute your exposure. You may be able to manage using the equipment for shorter chunks of time if you take breaks during which you move to one of the locations where you never experience symptoms.

Electrical Equipment in Today's Home

Room	Electrical Equipment			
Kitchen	Battery clock	Dishwasher	Freezer	Slow cooker
	Bread maker	Electric clock	Fridge	Sound system
	Can opener	Electronic scales	Microwave	Television
	Coffee/Tea maker	Extractor fan	Range	
	Dehydrator	Fluorescent light	Battery chargers for cordless appliances	
Bedroom	Air purifier	Cell phone charger	Electric blanket	Sound system
	Answering machine	Clock radio	Fan	Surge protector
	Automatic lights	Computer	Night light	Water bed
	Baby monitor	Dimmer switch	Printer	
	Battery clock	Battery chargers for remote controlled cars and cordless phone		
Bathroom	Electronic scales	Fluorescent light	Whirlpool tub	
	Fan	Heated towel rack	Battery chargers for toothbrushes and shavers	
Utility	Battery recharger	Fluorescent light	Sewing machine	Washer
	Dryer	Fan	Battery charger for cordless vacuum	
Workshop	Electric tools	Fluorescent light	Battery chargers for cordless power tools	
Family	Air conditioner	Cell phone charger	Electric heater	Television
	Air purifier	Computer	Printer	VCR
	Answering machine	Dimmer switch	Sound system	
	Automatic lights	DVD	Surge protector	
Office	Air purifier	Cell phone charger	Electric typewriter	Photocopier
	Answering machine	Computer	Fax machine	Printer
	Automatic lights	Dimmer Switch	Modem	Projector
				Surge protector
Other	Dog fence	Intercom	Security system	Smoke detector
	Garage door opener	Pest repeller	Carbon monoxide detector	

Step 8:

Restoring Balance

If your symptoms are related to your indoor environment, you will notice a change almost immediately as you implement the Simple Steps. Healing, however, takes time and the more careful you are to maintain minimal chemical and electromagnetic levels in your home, the faster your healing will proceed. There will still be occasions when your symptoms reappear, but when they do, look around you: what do you notice about your surroundings? Are you asking your body to cope with an environment it isn't yet well enough to deal with?

Physical

Your energy level may have been affected by the fact that you don't know what is wrong with you. Exercise, however, is an important part of getting your body back to normal functioning. Begin by walking for five minutes a day and increase the time to half an hour as you heal. Make sure that the route you walk is well away from any significant source of power — cell phone towers, power lines, substations, etc.

When you reach half an hour of walking, think back to the physical activities you enjoyed before you became sick. You may not be able to resume mountain climbing for a while, but maybe you enjoyed dancing, yoga, or an exercise class. Every effort you make to become involved in physical activity will contribute to your well-being.

Emotional

For a long time now, your main focus has been your health problems. You may well have alienated some people you cared about and find yourself isolated. You have to move on from here because the very fact that you have pursued the Simple Steps affirms the fact that you want your life and you want to live it fully. Many people have been where you are now and they will all tell you that, with a little more perseverance, you can pick up the pieces and move forward.

You know better than anyone what your emotional needs are. Think back to times in your life when you have been happy. You probably had purpose,

Worksheet 10: *Tracking Responses tp Electrical Appliances.* **Date:**

Instructions: Write the names of electrical appliances that are in use in your home at the heads of the columns. Keep a daily record of your use of each one, including the times when you turned it on and off. Record any reactions, including when they appeared and how long they lasted.

Symptoms:							
Monday							
Tuesday							
Wednesday							
Thursday							
Friday							
Saturday							
Sunday							

companionship, achievement, and satisfaction. Try to analyze what the things were that made you feel positive about yourself. Use these criteria to set yourself some small, achievable goals one week at a time.

Psychological

You've spent a long time preoccupied with your health concerns and your healing may not be as rapid as you would like it to be, considering the effort you have put into it. Set yourself some small goals. They may be as simple as making it to the next meal or being able to balance on one foot to the count of 10 with your eyes closed. Whatever your goals, make sure they are achievable — and reward your success.

Your preoccupation with your health has probably set you up for some ridicule and you may well feel alienated and alone. You may not have met your fellow sufferers, but be assured that you are most definitely not alone. We've all experienced the jokes at our expense — the husband who tells everyone that it's too stressful for you to do the dishes, the friend who tells everyone you've lost your marbles. People don't mean to be unkind — they just don't understand. Try to surround yourself with people who will bolster your spirits, people who are active and interesting to talk to, who laugh and listen.

You can increase your social interaction by participating in an activity with other people who have purpose — sitting around with other sick people won't do it for you, but enrolling in a pottery class might. Initially, you may not want to get involved in anything too demanding, but a little volunteering in an activity you enjoy may be just the reintroduction to society that you need.

You may have lost track of time in your period of worry, and now that days are back to normal, it is important to make sure that you follow a structure. Eat your meals at regular times and plan your morning, afternoon, and evening activities. Don't make your plans too ambitious because you need to be able to stick to the activities you have selected. Reward your achievement. Make sure that at least one time slot in each day contains an activity that brings you into contact with other people.

Use Worksheet 11 to help plan your day. Four copies will keep you going for your first month. As it is impossible to predict how long it will take to restore a balanced state of health, you may need to keep using a daily plan for some time, so make sure you keep one blank copy of the worksheet on hand.

Try to plan your activities at least a day ahead, and include one activity each day that involves interaction with healthy people. An activity that repeats weekly can take care of several chunks of time — for instance, the book club at the library, a drawing class (but avoid any location where painting also takes place), or, depending on your state of health, a fitness class. As you check out what is available, make sure that you can tolerate the location before you sign up. Record enough about your meals to make sure they are regular. Write down your weekly goals and successes. One of your greatest sources of encouragement may come from comparing the worksheet from the previous week — and noting how much more you managed to accomplish this week.

You will know when you are ready to move out of your sanctuary, but when you do, be careful to move to a bed where your sleep is undisturbed. You will probably have to change the position of your bed. Try it in several positions before deciding which is best and then rearrange the other furniture.

Chemicals and electromagnetic fields will creep back into your environment as you get better. A periodic review of the worksheets will help you to maintain your compatible environment. Don't be afraid to let a few sources of chemicals and electromagnetic fields become part of your day, but do maintain the minimal EMF environment at night.

Continue with your new diet. But you give yourself a little slack — the odd McDonald's or other processed food can be a welcome addition to your meals, but keep them in check. When the Canada Food Guide sets up its food groups, it really is talking about the foods that appear on the pictures — not the ones that they are processed into.

It took me an awfully long time to recover once I had implemented all my strategies; even when the symptoms stopped, my immune system remained weak for a good six months. My return to the health I now enjoy took the better part of a year. Today, I remain aware of the dangers that electricity and chemicals have for me. I watch their entry into my home with a scrutiny based on the knowledge that there is a deep, dark, frightening cave to which I will not return.

Worksheet 11: *Daily Plan to Restore Balance.*   **Date:**

Instructions: Structure your day in advance. Plan an achieveable activity for each time period. At least one activity each day should be spent in the company of healthy, positive people. Set yourself an achievable goal for the week, and choose a reward when you are successful.

	Morning Breakfast at	**Afternoon** Lunch at	**Evening** Dinner at
Monday			
Tuesday			
Wednesday			
Thursday			
Friday			
Saturday			
Sunday			
This week's goal is…			
Rewards for success are…			

Part Three

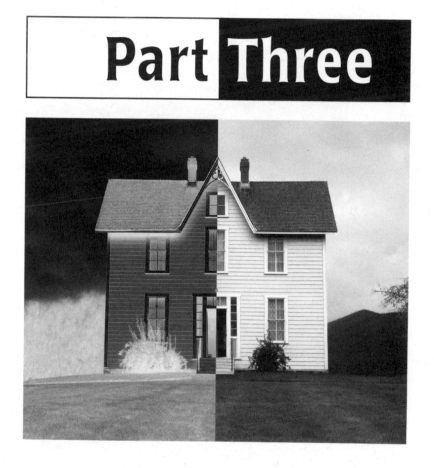

Case Studies: Can You Spot the Danger?

O NE OF THE MAIN DIFFICULTIES WITH THE SYMPTOMS OF INDOOR POLLUTION is that when we go to the doctor's office looking for help, the symptoms don't come with us. With the insight gained so far into the sources of indoor pollution, can you spot the dangers lurking in the following case studies? If you can, you may find that you can give your doctor a great deal more information about your symptoms when you next find yourself turning to him for help. Often we describe our symptoms to the doctor, expecting him to tell us what is wrong from across the desk. We don't realize that from the other side of the desk, the doctor can only work with the information we give him. He can't see the symptoms as the effect of common mistakes and advise us how to fix the mistakes. All he can do is match the symptoms with chemical remedies.

A Day in the Life

"Jimmy"

Jimmy gets up in the morning. He climbs down from his space-saving bunk to answer his cordless phone. He checks his e-mail on the computer. Both the phone and the computer are on his desk under his bed. He gets washed and dresses in chemically-softened, peach-scented clothes. He sits down to his cereal enriched with vitamins and laced with neuron-compromising flavor enhancers and coal tar. He goes off to school. At school he learns about the dangers of smoking, alcohol, and drugs while seated below the school's cell

> **!**
> Did you know that pediatricians in America were only recently alerted to the possible evironmental causes of children's symptoms with the distribution of a "Handbook of Pediatric Environmental Health?"[1]

phone tower. For lunch he eats his pizza pockets and Jell-O, and spends recess playing under the power lines that cross the school playground. After school Jimmy heads home. He grabs a Coke and a cookie and sits down to play Nintendo with his face inches away from the screen. He grabs his battery pack from the permanently-plugged-in battery charger below his bed and goes off to play with his remote control car. Do you recognize Jimmy? Isn't he the same child who is doing the rounds of the doctors with his frantic mother trying to find answers and help for his seizures, allergies, asthma, and persistent bronchitis?

Jimmy has been on anti-convulsive medication for years. He spends some five hours a day playing Nintendo with his face inches from the screen and then goes off to bed to sleep with his head just inches from where the power comes into the house from the transformer above his bedroom window. He's a picky eater who's allowed to eat cereal all day if he wants to because "at least then he's eating something."

Do you recognize the danger spots in Jimmy's environment — the computer, power pack, and battery charger under his bed, the lack of any real nutrition, the abundance of chemicals, the transformer above his head, etc.? We almost want to scream, because now it is all so obvious to us. But if we did try to tell Jimmy's mother to look at these hazards she would say, "I'll ask the doctor." The doctor would say, "Jimmy needs to be on anti-convulsive medication because he has seizures." So Jimmy continues to suffer and though the medication controls the seizures, its side effects give him that classic "out to lunch look," make him inaccessible to his peers, and prevent him getting it together enough to do his school work What would it cost the adults to try just once to take his environment into consideration? And what would it give Jimmy if it worked?

With all the chemicals and EMFs that we add to our home environments — far, far more than existed when we were children — it seems almost basic to consider them in relation to our ailments rather than waiting to outgrow them. Children interact with their environment three times as much as adults for their body weight.[2] We start them off at three months with their first dose of mercury in vaccinations, many of which are available in mercury-free preparations. We continue with regular doses of vaccinations until our children are five years old. We offer another dose when they are eleven in our efforts to protect them from hepatitis and extra doses anywhere in between to protect against various strains of meningitis. We

> Did you know that ethyl mercuri thiosalicyclic acid, an organic mercury compound commonly referred to as thimerosol, is the most widely used preservative in vaccines —and that we give it to our infants before they begin to make the bile they need to excrete it?[4]

feed them on cereals and fast food laced with flavor enhancers known to cause neuron damage.[3] We dress them in more new clothes than adults wear because they grow out of them. With each new article of clothing their little bodies have to deal with mercury residues from the dyes and an abundance of chemicals from the sizing — and that's assuming that we don't swath them in fabrics that are made from chemicals in the first place. With our new wrinkle-releasing sprays and air fresheners we can even add an extra layer of chemicals. To top it all off, we march them off to the dentist for their annual dose of radiation in the form of x-rays to check for cavities.

While mothers and fathers search through conventional and traditional medicine for medications that will relieve their symptoms, their children's immune systems continue to be compromised by the very environments they create for them. While the parents fill another prescription for Ritalin and antibiotics and reach for the cough mixture, the children crawl back into their beds surrounded by the electronic trappings of the twenty-first century (all of them electrically powered over night!) with their tummies full of pre-prepared, chemically-laced, fast "foods."

"Stephanie"

Stephanie came home from the hospital two days old, welcomed by her eager family. In her honor, all the air fresheners had been refilled, the nursery freshly painted, and the new crib adorned with new, unwashed, polyester bumper pads and a matching polyester quilt. Her loving parents had gone to the expense of acquiring the latest baby monitor that had a pad under the sheet to sense her movements, an electric mobile, a dimmer switch on the light, and a closet full of little dresses.

How many newborns come home to an environment just like this? And how many of them adapt and thrive? Stephanie didn't. Within a week she was back at the doctor's office, covered from head to toe in a rash, crying endlessly and feeding poorly. The doctor faulted the mother's milk and Stephanie was put on soy formula — all of which, in Canada, is genetically altered.

Another week passed: Stephanie was put on antibiotics for her bronchitis; a week later she was hospitalized because of breathing difficulties; and for the rest of her first year, she was in and out of hospital several times. As the time approached for her to begin eating solid food, she frequently came out in rashes, vomited, and had endless diarrhea. Her well-meaning parents added a humidifier to her nursery and kept the air fresheners topped up to help cover the smell of Stephanie's constant sickness; they invested in an electric rocker to try to soothe her, and bathed her in every product that claimed to be soothing. But whatever they did, Stephanie continued to be a sickly child: no matter what electrical appliance or chemical concoction they added to her environment, nothing seemed to give her any relief. Desperate for answers and help, they looked to allergists and naturopaths, but everywhere they turned the health professionals diagnosed another allergy — until eventually little Stephanie was allergic to dust, nuts, wheat, and lactose. What really worried her parents was that even when they avoided these products, Stephanie remained sickly.

Do you recognize the danger spots? Are the hazards as obvious to you now as they could possibly be? Have you noticed all the chemicals in Stephanie's environment and all the sources of electromagnetic fields? Do you just want to scream at the doctors and the parents to tell them that none of their dietary changes or creams have cured Stephanie? Do you want to alert them to the possibility that they may indeed be creating an incompatible environment by focusing their efforts to find a cure on adding something rather than taking something away?

Throughout their pregnancies, mothers-to-be pray for a healthy baby — a child who won't be hampered in his development by anything that we could have prevented. We sue mightily when other people's negligence undermines the promise of our children, yet we bring them into home environments where their daily exposure will have a longer and more profound impact on their health than many of the things we feared.

When my children were born their pediatrician recommended that I soothe my crying infant by putting his bassinet on the dryer or next to the vacuum cleaner: the white noise and the gentle hum would soothe him to sleep. Was it really the sound and vibrations that had calmed him? Or had the EMF from these appliances affected his body as they did mine? If EMFs could knock me out at 130 pounds, then what could they do to a ten-pound baby? Since EMFs affect the hormones that regulate the heart and vascular system,[6] what chance does a baby have?

> Did you know that a 1999 study found that mice exposed to disposable diapers suffered eye, nose, and throat irritations? The "superabsorbents" found in diapers were withdrawn from use in tampons in 1980.[5]

How many of today's sick children cannot handle the environments we create for them? How many of us recognize the hazards posed by polyester bumper pads and bedding, carcinogenic talc, chlorine-bleached, chemically-laden diapers, chemically-softened clothes, baby monitors, electronic kicking toys, electric mobiles, and genetically altered soy formula? We've become so accustomed to trying new things that we don't even notice the build-up of chemicals. We'd never consider storing a bottle of screen wash or bleach in the nursery, even on a high shelf, but the chemicals are the same!

"Fred and Joe"

Fred is always sick; he catches every cold at the office, suffers from migraines and rashes, and is allergic to cats. Joe on the other hand, never has a cold, can count his headaches on one hand, and doesn't understand why Fred keeps kicking his cat. At first sight, Fred and Joe appear to live similar lives: they get up and jog in the morning, drive an hour to work, spend part of the evening watching television, and set their alarms as they turn in for the night. On closer

> **!** Did you kow that all the soy used in baby formula in Canada is genetically altered, though in Europe, genetically-altered, soy-based infant formula is banned because of health effects?[7]

inspection, we can see a huge difference between their personal environments.

Fred takes his morning jog down the main street under the power-lines breathing in exhaust fumes. He showers, dresses in his dry-cleaned suit, and sets off in his Honda Odyssey. The huge EMFs from the disk brakes soon put pins and needles in his feet, and he stops to grab a coke and a donut from the drive-through fast-food outlet. Revived, he continues his stressful hour-long drive under power lines to work. Here he takes his place at his computer. The carefully designed office provides partitions to aid concentration, which results in the computers being set back to back. For lunch, Fred grabs a coffee and a burger and completes his day with a couple of very stressful meetings. Fred drives home under the power lines, heats a pre-prepared meal, and plays a couple of computer games. Before he settles down for the remainder of the evening, inches from a large screen TV, he changes the plug in an air freshener that makes the smell of his feet bearable. As the day ends, he crawls into his bed, located inches from the power entry to the condos. He reaches up to set his digital alarm, plugs in his cell-phone to recharge it, and turns over in the hope of a good night's sleep.

Joe lives three doors down from Fred in the same development. He takes his morning jog through the park where the air is sweet and no power lines obscure the view. He showers, dresses in his dry-cleaned suit which has been aired because he doesn't like the smell of dry cleaning, then sits down to juice and bagels. He climbs into his manual Honda Civic with its low EMFs, and drives the quiet way to work; he doesn't mind that it takes an extra five minutes, because it's less stressful than the main drag. When Joe gets to the office, he greets Fred and sits down at his computer, located along the outside wall. For lunch, Joe brings a hearty sandwich from home. He joins Fred for the afternoon meetings; they're a breeze to him. When the day ends, Joe drives home along his favorite route. He stops for a while to read his book in the park, then goes home to cook himself some supper — a baked potato, a homemade burger, with a generous salad and a glass of filtered water. A couple more chapters of his book and a television program finish off his day and he winds up his manual alarm clock as he gets into bed. He has no cell phone to plug in because he finds the availability they imply stressful.

On first appearance Fred and Joe appear to live pretty normal lives and we could be forgiven for thinking that they live in the same environment; they work in the same office and live in the same condo. But on closer inspection we see a huge difference in their personal environments: Fred and Joe's radiation exposure is significantly different. Fred has surrounded himself with significant sources of EMFs during both the day and night — from the power lines, the van, his co-workers' computers, the TV, the power to the building, the cell phone recharger, and the digital alarm clock. Fred's chemical load is also significantly higher than Joe's; he starts off with exhaust and dry-cleaning fumes, and consumes chemically-laden foods. Were he experiencing any uncomfortable symptoms, he would do well to consider this exposure. With so much interference, his hormones may be struggling to go about their business efficiently, leaving his immune system overloaded before Joe's cat walks in. Joe's radiation exposure on the other hand is far less constant and much lower. Only his own computer has caused any interference to his hormones and his immune system is able to measure up to the day's onslaughts. It won't matter how much Fred sneezes at him, he won't get sick.

"Theresa, Mary, and Shelley"

Theresa has two daughters. Since they moved into their house by the power lines, Shelley has been suffering with psoriasis while Mary has outbursts and vicious headaches. Not knowing anything about the effect of power lines and maybe having too great a stake in her house to find anything out, Theresa marches her children off to the doctor on a regular basis. The doctor prescribes creams for the psoriasis and considers Ritalin for the inattention that Shelley has shown since a cell phone tower was installed on the school roof.

So why is the mother fine in this same environment? Theresa has made the same assumption that so many of us make. If the symptoms were provoked by an external stimulus, then everyone would be sick. If some people are well in the same environment, the sick person must be suffering from an internal disease.

On closer inspection, though, we soon see that the immediate environment of each of these family members differs significantly. Theresa's bedroom is at the back of the house, away from the power lines, while the girls share a room at the front of the house, much closer to the power lines. They have a computer in their bedroom which they leave on all day, partly because their picture is on the screen saver and partly because they feel it takes a long time to start it. Because it is always on, the computer is plugged into a surge protector. Mary's bed broke, so her mattress is on the floor which puts her head less than a foot above the smoke detector on the living room ceiling.

When they sit down to breakfast, Theresa toasts herself a bagel while Mary and Shelley start the day with bowls of Fruit Loops and milk. As the girls head off to school, mum gets the laundry done. Shelley's cotton clothes are carefully rinsed because of her psoriasis. Mary's clothes are dried with a Downy sheet so they'll smell fresh longer.

At school Shelley heads for her classroom, a temporary addition with recently-glued carpets. The smell greets her as far away as the bathroom; she retches and wishes she could go home, but there'd be so much catching up to do. She's relieved when the teacher leaves the door open; if only the window wasn't sealed shut.

Mary joins her class below the cell phone tower and takes her seat next to the six new computers and their surge protectors which they need because they'll be on all day. Like her sister, she wishes the windows weren't sealed; everything smells so bad!

Both girls get some respite from the smells as they walk home under the power lines to have their lunch. Mum has a whole grain sandwich and makes Mary a hot-dog because she doesn't want the pizza that Shelley is having. They all drink sodas and the girls head back to school for the afternoon. Mary takes a couple of Tylenol first, because her head hurts so much.

We could be flies on the wall for the rest of the day, but I think we can see already just how different the immediate environment of each family member is. We can already see what the doctors can't and we already want to move Mary's bed. If we were asked for help we know we would ventilate those classrooms, and put those computers somewhere else to offgas. We know we would remove the surge protectors with their high EMFs and remove the cell phone tower. We would add some foods bursting with nutrients — foods that didn't contain preservatives or colors. We can see that without the knowledge of these seemingly innocuous hazards in our immediate environments, the doctor doesn't get the full picture. Without an understanding of the complete picture, these children can be doomed to years of needless medication and suffering.

Failure of Conventional Medical Solutions

Most of us deal with sickness the way we were taught as children: we keep warm, stay out of draughts, take a couple of Tylenol, and rest. If our symptoms persist we try another over-the-counter remedy, and if they persist beyond that, we go to the doctor for something a bit stronger. We may get something from the doctor that fixes us the first time, but we may have to go back and have the prescription changed in some way. When we do hit on a drug that relieves our symptoms, we like our doctors, consider ourselves cured. In our reliance on pharmaceutical companies, we rarely stop to consider that the drug industry thrives on our belief in a "pill for every ill." It seldom occurs to us that preventing disease benefits only the patient; we rarely question how many medical charities are sustained by our belief in a cure around the corner.[8]

Our society accepts illness as an inevitability. We know that one in eight women will get breast cancer and one in eight men will get prostate cancer; we hope we'll be among the seven who don't. We know one in twelve people suffer from migraines and hope that we'll be among the eleven that don't.

We take great comfort from our belief that someone is out there looking for a cure; we are reassured by the very act of sealing the envelope that contains our contribution to research. It rarely occurs to us that we might be looking to the wrong people for solutions. It seems absurd that we should expect solutions from the very industry that created the problem: even Einstein warned against this. Yet isn't that exactly what we're expecting from industries that produce devices that emit EMFs?

Secure in our faith in pharmaceutical cures, we watch our children grow. We hope they will be healthy, but accept the possibility they will be amongst the unlucky ones who suffer from allergies, asthma, migraines, and seizures. If they are, we will give them something to relieve their symptoms and eliminate anything known to provoke their symptoms. But what if, like me, they have tested positive to allergens that are not associated with their symptoms? With ten percent of Canadian children suffering from asthma and a 100 percent increase in peanut allergies in the last ten years, at what point do we begin to wonder if maybe there is something preying on their developing systems making them more vulnerable to these allergens? Why is it that in one school there are ten children who carry EpiPens for anaphylactic shock reactions and in others there are none? How can peanut products be banned in some schools while others have never heard of peanut allergies? Can we be sure that we're looking for answers in the right places?

The Chemical "Cure"

The change from healing as an art that involved the balancing of the mind, body, and spirit began with Fleming's discovery of penicillin. He was one of the first to make the suggestion that symptoms could be balanced by chemical concoctions. The financial incentive to the inventors of successful drugs, and profits for the drug companies that produce them, provided the encouragement that made this one branch of medicine grow out of all proportion to the rest. Today's belief in a pill for every ill is the result of this unbalanced growth. We no longer look around us; we no longer make connections between our symptoms and the changes we have made to our immediate environments. We're not prepared to consider that Sam has been getting more colds since we started using air fresheners, or that Mary's recent sensitivity to animals may be influenced by the new position of her bed directly above the fuse box. Our recent anxiety attacks couldn't possibly be related to the high EMFs from the new car's disk brakes.

Sharks – Seeing the Whole Picture

Our commitment to the philosophy of a pill for every ill skews our vision of the larger picture, causing us to miss some of the most valuable information we have. Take, for example, the development of the use of shark cartilage in the fight against cancer. Since sharks only rarely get cancer, researchers suspect there must be something in their cartilage that prevents the development of blood vessels to tumors. In an effort to create a drug that might pass the shark's capacity to avoid cancer to humans, shark cartilage is ground up and used for its anti-angiogenesis capabilities. As yet this remedy is only available in herbal medicine but efforts are being made to get FDA approval.[9]

Looking for something that can be ground up into the next wonder drug, the researchers may have missed the most crucial part of the picture — that sharks sense EMFs and swim away from them. Though it may be their cartilage that doesn't allow for the growth of tumors, could it not also be that their simple immune systems are enhanced by their intense sensitivity to EMFs and their consequent ability to avoid areas where EMFs would interfere with their bodies' systems and make them sick?

Though we might not see the whole picture, we can see enough of it to work out a way to swim with the sharks. A device was recently introduced which exploits the sharks' ability to sense EMFs, enabling divers to swim with them. Now divers can swim in shark-infested waters, even hand feed the sharks, with these devices in packs strapped on their backs. If the shark gets too excited, the diver can push a button and surround himself with EMFs. The sharks know to get away from the source of EMFs, but we strap it to our backs!

If we looked at the whole picture we might be able to see these sharks in the same light as the canaries that were once used to warn coal miners of dangerous gases in the mines. The Round Gobi fish, too, with their sensitivity to EMFs, might hold some answers for us. Like sharks they avoid EMFs — an ability that is exploited in our efforts to keep them out of the Mississippi. Almost all of the fish turn back when they hit the EMF barrier.[10]

> Did you know that even the fruit fly drosophila makes an effort to lay her eggs away from EMFs? When she doesn't succeed, the eggs laid in EMFs have a significantly lower survival rate than those not exposed.[11]

"Take Something" or "Take Something Away"?

Had the development of medicine achieved the balance we would like to think it stands for, maybe environmental considerations would have more weight in current practice. We might not consider them only as a last resort, or expect balance to be restored by drugs. We might not be surprised to find our doctors telling us to unplug our air fresheners, or suggesting we look at our immediate environments before considering drug therapies. I suspect we would all be more adept at identifying the hazards in our immediate environments, recognizing when an immune system was taking a beating, working out the causes, and removing the burdens. Prevention would be key, just as it is when we think about safety.

When we have learned to take preventative measures, they tend be to in the form of avoiding sick people, or boosting our immune systems by taking things such as echinacea. But taking something to boost our immune systems isn't terribly far removed from the premise of a pill for every ill. Though echinacea goes a long way to boosting the immune system in an otherwise balanced body and can enable our bodies to stop colds dead in their tracks, the measures we take to heal the unbalanced body have to be more intense. For those people whose symptoms may be attributable to provocative agents in their environments, we have to think not simply in terms of taking something but in terms of taking something away. Taking something to ease their symptoms has to take a back seat to isolating and removing the burdens in their individual environments.

It seems ironic that, because of our trust in medication, we ignore the environment in which our symptoms occur. More often than not, the victims of sick houses are told that their symptoms are psychosomatic and they are returned to the very environment that provoked their symptoms — places where they can only continue to deteriorate.

When only one person in our midst is sick, we need to consider the exposures in their immediate environment. Even amongst members of a family, the immediate environment of each person living in the same house is different. Each individual's interaction with his immediate environment is personal. Each person sleeps in his own pocket of EMF, and consumes his own combination of chemicals in his air, food, and water. This total interaction plays a role in defining a person's health. When we recognize that environments are specific to the individual, and we can point very specifically to their burdens, it suddenly ceases to be as difficult as it was to create compatible environments for them. We can help them make connections — connections that will enable them to live their lives to the full.

Modifying Our Understanding of Health

Our unwillingness to consider our health in relation to the environment we create for ourselves leaves us susceptible to a whole range of avoidable symptoms and drugs. The belief that radiation from our electrical devices is limited to the vicinity of the appliance, our faith in safety levels for chemicals, and the presence of so many healthy people sharing the same environment make it difficult to think that our symptoms are anything but the expression of internal disease.

Even globally, there is an unwillingness to consider the rise in allergies, asthma, MS, Alzheimer's, Parkinson's, depression, autism, learning disabilities, and certain cancers in relation to EMFs — yet they present the single biggest concurrent increase in pollution in the civilized world. Since Edison's bright idea in 1880, the amount of electricity flowing to our homes has steadily increased. In addition to the twenty-fold increase in the use of electricity since 1940, we must now add the EMFs emitted by our cell phones and wireless communications. As we buy more things to protect, we need more systems to protect them. With houses built closer together, the layering effect of all these EMFs is increased.

Warnings from concerned researchers about the dangers of EMFs are quickly discredited by the stronger voices of industry. We listen to these loud voices as they tell us that "The dangers have not yet been proven"; "Animal studies can't tell us what we need to know about humans"; "Without new technologies we can't maximize efficiency"; or "Our decisions must be based on 'sound science'." We seem more willing to listen to the industry's argument than to the warnings. But maybe Lloyds of London has good reason to refuse to insure cell phone companies against the damage to their buyers.[12] Maybe we depend on animal research for much of our information, and maybe if there weren't so many impediments, some of the theories on the health effects of EMFs could move into the realms of sound science. Rather than heed the warnings, we take the risks!

If we recognize the possibility that EMFs and chemicals in the quantities we use them add a burden to our bodies that weakens them, just what are we prepared to do about it? Would we take Jimmy's computer out of his room, would we impose rules that no phone or battery chargers are to be used at night? Can we force Jimmy to take a sandwich and juice for lunch, or are we concerned that he will appear less than cool to his peers? Could we open the windows in Stephanie's room and remove the chemicals and air freshener? Would we feel safe if we removed the monitor from under her mattress? Even if we accept that environmental factors chip away at our bodies, even if we accept that we would be better off if we removed some of the offending sources, are we prepared to remove them? Can we accept the stripping away of a luxury we've become accustomed to having, as a way of giving our bodies a break? Can we imagine ourselves saying, "Tonight I'm going to give my body a break. I'm not going to slide into that bubble bath – my immune system is getting the night off."

EMFs in Our Communities:

What We Can Do to Mitigate the Dangers

I N MANY ASPECTS OF OUR SOCIETY, situations change long before the rules that govern them. Just as we think everything is under control, our intellectual and creative talents take us to new heights. As contexts change, we create new rules and standards — but the contexts change first.

The technological changes that we have witnessed in the last forty years — and the difficulties we have keeping regulations and safety standards in line with that change — are a prime illustration of this phenomenon. Where once our bright, tangential thinkers would have been drawn to scientific research, today they are drawn to the world of the technological industries where their creative talents and vision are appreciated. In no time at all, they and their companies are catapulted into fame and fortune, and from there, they direct the research into electromagnetic fields and health. The very things that dissuaded them from the path of non-profit research — restrictions, the need for reproducible results, battles with orthodox schools of thought, and the huge gap between discovery and the acceptance of their findings into the realm of orthodox science — become their allies as they reach for the stars. While researchers follow a line of inquiry that may have no concrete results, the bright minds in the corporate world provide their customers with tangible products that appeal to our society's sense of progress. As consumers, we resist the suggestion that the by-products of technology might be bad for us. Research scientists have been diligently warning us for years that EMFs have an adverse impact on our health, but such warnings threaten the continuing growth of our technological

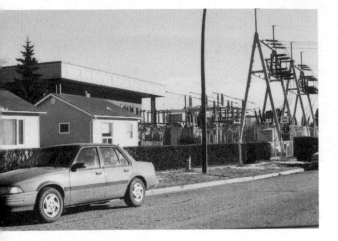

*Above: Danger in the Neighborhood. People living in homes located near strong sources of EMFs are highly likely to experience a multitude of health complaints. The standards governing safe levels of exposure were developed when the electrical demands of the average home were minimal. **Below**: Danger in the Backyard.*
***Credit**: Angela Hobbs.*

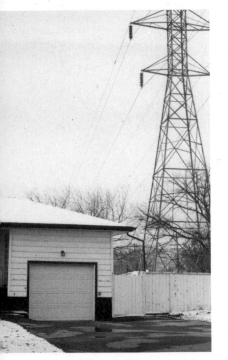

industries. We need to ask: what good is technological progress if it makes us sick?

Power Lines

As our demand for electricity increases, power companies often push more current down existing wires until the new demand can justify building more distribution networks. When more electricity in pushed down a wire than it is designed to carry, the amount that is wasted along the way increases. This wasted electricity along the length of the wire adds to the already high levels of EMFs channeled over playgrounds, schools, and residences.[1]

Even at normal demand, before any "pushing" begins, the big wires that come from the power plants where electricity is generated carry 500 kilovolts. These wires are supported on the pylons that march through the countryside demanding clear-cut paths through the forest. They are the same pylons that cows cluster around in a daze. When the current reaches a major substation, the electricity in these wires is transformed to either 115 kilovolts or 230 kilovolts. This new current is then carried through our cities on primary distribution lines to local substations. The wires leaving the local substations carry currents of 4000 to 13,800 volts to the cylinders on posts or the little green boxes on our front lawns and in many of our gardens. Here they are downsized again to 120 or 240 volts and sent off into our houses.[2]

Land with power lines tends to be cheaper: the pylons are deemed unsightly and many people are skeptical of their safety. Schools, churches, and community organizations take advantage of the availability of this cheap land, with the result that children spend large amounts of time in places that can do them the most harm. Some children spend their whole day in classrooms 100 feet away from power lines. This is the "safe" distance according to Canada's Safety Code Six — a code founded on the belief that EMFs will only have biological effects if they cause heating. When our children fidget, we reprimand them and seek out drugs to help them concentrate.

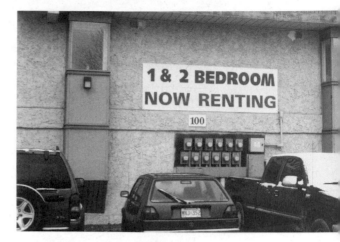

Alternatives

Decreasing our consumption of electricity would seem an obvious alternative to increasing distribution. The possibility of burying power lines in oil tubes is also an alternative, though without the oil, power lines underground actually cause higher EMFs at ground level than when the lines are overhead. Changing the configurations of the wires inside power lines is also an alternative. Both alternatives are expensive and also have an impact on transmission efficiency, so power companies have no incentive to make these changes — unless governments update safety standards.

My own children attend a school almost exactly 100 feet from a power line that delivers electricity from a substation to green box transformers. On damp nights the power line can be heard hissing and crackling as moisture amplifies the corona effect. I take solace in knowing that the children only spend six hours a day at school, that the computers and their

Above: Danger in the Apartment. Electricity for all twelve apartments in this building in Calgary, Alberta, passes through this wall. Occupants may be spending hours on a bed or sofa next to this area of high exposure to EMFs. **Credit**: *Angela Hobbs.*

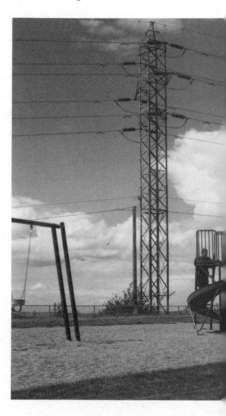

Left: Out of the Frying Pan, Into the Fire. Children taking breaks from computers and video games seek the fresh air of playgrounds. When playgrounds are located on cheap land under power lines, like this one in Calgary, Alberta, the exposure to EMFs that accompanies the fresh air can seriously affect the children's developing bodies. **Credit**: *Angela Hobbs.*

surge protectors are located in a separate room, and that the children know not to play under the power lines at recess. I also know that during the time that they are not at school the children are in an environment that is low in toxicity and EMF exposure.

Cell Phones

The convenience of the cell phone is undeniable. It's wonderful to be able to call anyone, anytime, anywhere; the additional cost of our phone bills is worth every penny. It is estimated that by 2005 there will be of 1.6 billion cell phones worldwide.[3]

When we take note of the downside of cell phones, it tends to be in terms of the danger they cause in traffic. Who hasn't noticed how blocked the left lane has become and how no one ever uses turn signals? We may take note of the impact that a cell phone base station will have on our view, but normally we have little interest in the health concerns raised by the prevalence of cell phones and their base stations.

Whether or not cell phones cause cancer isn't really the issue here — we know that the pulsed microwaves penetrate our bodies. We know that we can use microwaves to cook chickens and get supper in a hurry, so whatever effect they have, it can't be doing us much good. Microwaves add a burden to our bodies: for the cell phone user, the burden is from the near field where much of the electromagnetic energy is absorbed by the head, causing an increase in the brain's temperature. The harder the cell phone has to work to receive its signal, the greater the radiation it produces. For the rest of the population, the exposure is in the far field where the intensity varies depending on our distance from the base station, the number of communications it maintains, and the position of reflectors and directors relative to the antennae. The effects of the exposure in both the near and far field include radiofrequency sickness, changes in blood pressure, and cancer risks.[4]

Alternatives

Cell phones don't have to be an all-or-nothing issue if we take some informed action. One means of mitigating the risks to the user is the earpiece, which keeps the microwaves away from the head. Complemented with the use of voice-activated dialers, these developments also help to keep the driver's hands on the steering wheel.

Safety standards around the world differ significantly. For example, the safety standards for one cell phone frequency — 900 megahertz (MHz) — is lowest in Russia and Switzerland. Their public exposure limit is 2.4 microwatts per square centimeter ($\mu W/cm^2$). China's is three times higher at 6.6 $\mu W/cm^2$. Italy's limit is over forty times the Russian limit at 100 $\mu W/cm^2$. And the limit of the International Commission on Non-Ionizing Radiation Protection (ICNIRP) used almost everywhere else, including North America, is 200 times the Russian limit at 450 $\mu W/cm^2$.[5]

Cell Phone Transmitters

In order to have the option of picking up a cell phone, transmitter base stations have to be erected to service them. The rapid proliferation of these base stations would put any rabbit to shame. Many are erected on schools and on churches — both the schools and churches can gain a great deal of revenue from them.

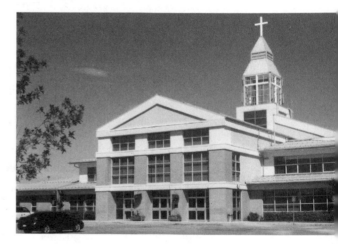

Cell phone companies want us to think that these base stations are directional; that their signal only goes in a specified direction. Some of them may, but most of them don't, because what good would they be if the signal was limited? Would we want a cell phone that we could only use in certain locations? Wouldn't that defeat the purpose? In either case, it takes time before the direction is focused which means that in the immediate vicinity of the base station, the signal pretty much permeates in all directions, unhampered by roofs, walls or ceilings. While we're at church services and our children are at preschool in the church basement or at

*Cell Phone Companies Pay For Church Towers. Church towers attract cell phone companies because they can provide the height required for cell phone transmitters. Congregations can gain substantial revenue from tower rentals; sometimes the cell phone company actually donates the cost of building a spire, as happened in this church in Calgary, Alberta. Unsuspecting parishioners and their children are exposed to high levels of EMFs while attending services and activities. **Credit**: Angela Hobbs.*

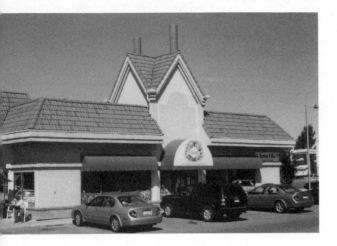

*Above: Can You Spot the Cell Phone Tower? **Below:** What's On Top of This Pole? The average passerby in Calgary, Alberta, may notice the unusual chimneys on this coffee shop and the odd pole topping this mall sign but few may realize that both are cell phone towers in disguise. **Credit:** Angela Hobbs.*

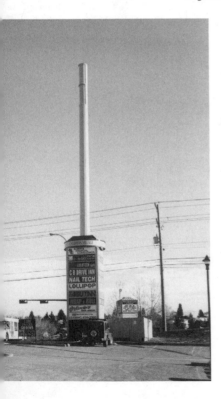

public school under a base station, we are all cocooned in their microwaves.

Alternatives

Situating base stations away from buildings where people live and work seems an obvious solution — one that more and more communities are opting for. If cell phone companies shared transmitters, fewer would be needed. The illustration on page 145 (Location of Cell Phone Transmitters of Competing Companies) shows how cell phone companies, each of whom have their own transmitters, create a significant amount of traffic in the air around us. The second illustration (Cell Phone Transmitters Required When Companies Collaborate) shows how much less traffic there would be if cell phone companies worked on a shared system — similar to the way traditional telephone companies share long distance cables. The number of transmitters would be lower and the overall field would be significantly smaller. Services would be as good as ever and total field strength would increase only as capacity needs demanded it. Defining complete coverage would set a limit on the number of base stations needed. Despite complete cell phone coverage of the city, another seventy base stations were licensed in Calgary in 2001.

Italy leads the world as the first country to draw up legislation preventing base stations from being built on schools and populated buildings. Where they are present and their fields exceed 20 volts per meter or 6 volts per meter for exposure for more than four hours, there is recourse. People caught in these situations have a right to free measurement of the exposure to EMFs and to request the removal of the base station.

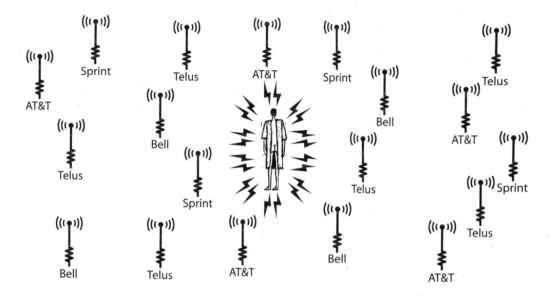

Above: Cell Phone Transmitters as Located by Competing Companies. *Below*: Cell Phone Transmitters Required When Companies Collaborate.

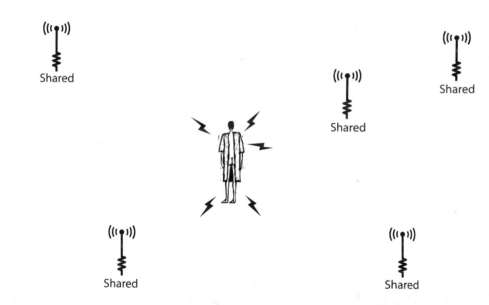

In Australia, the state of New South Wales has been working with a policy since 1997 of a 500 meter-radius corridor around base stations. Within this radius, there can be no schools, residences, nursing homes, hospitals, or

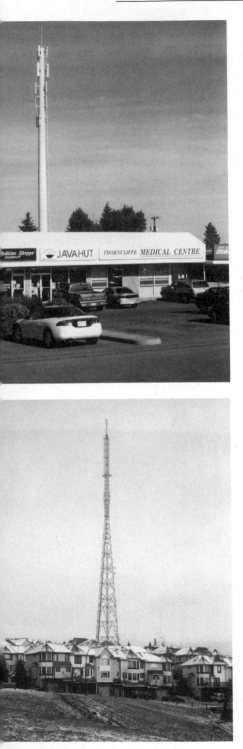

daycare centers. Where base stations already existed, efforts have been made to change their location.

Where no regulations exist, efforts by communities to create a moratorium on the building of base stations on schools, residences, hospitals, daycare centers, and nursing homes have been unsuccessful. On the whole, the concern of authorities remains one of appearance rather than safety. In the United Kingdom, telecommunication companies don't need the consent of the local authority to build base stations less than 15 meters high. In my own community in Calgary, Alberta, the only thing stopping the construction of a base station on our 1400-acre park is its unsightly appearance.

The relative youth of the cell phone industry means that many of the base stations that will be needed have not yet been built. In the United States, only 15 percent of planned cell phone base stations had been activated by the year 2001. It would seem to make a lot of sense to establish a regulation governing a clear distance between base stations and the places where people spend extended periods of time. Without the implementation of some safety measures to limit our exposure to base stations, the price that we actually pay for the luxury of cell phones will be far higher than the amount on our bills. While we wait for the legislation to be made, our children may be educated on the dangers of drugs and alcohol but they are unprotected from microwaves radiating down from the base stations above their heads.

Above: Not So Healthy a Center. Doctors and pharmacists who set up practice below cell phone towers, as in this mall in Calgary, Alberta, may not be knowledgeable about symptoms provoked by such an environment. Below: Broadcasting EMFs. This television transmitter in Calgary, Alberta, bathes the unsuspecting community at its base in EMFs all day and night Credit: Angela Hobbs.

Broadcasting Transmitters

Broadcasting transmitters for television and radio produce huge levels of EMFs. People who work at broadcasting studios are as vulnerable as air traffic engineers and controllers in their susceptibility to cancers and other diseases. The unsuspecting workers are engulfed in electromagnetic energy day after day. The more access we want to radio and TV, the more transmitters and relays are needed to service our luxury. The more transmitters there are, the more likely they are to be located close to our homes.

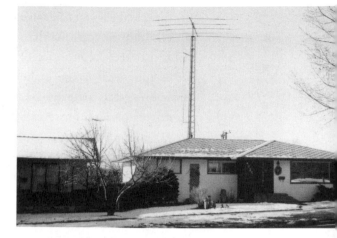

Above: *Ham Operators Broadcast EMFs from Home. The signals broadcast by amateur radio enthusiasts can greatly exceed the EMFs generated by cell phone transmitters. Unsuspecting neighbors in this Calgary suburb may find themselves running to their doctors with unusual symptoms.* **Credit**: *Angela Hobbs.*

Alternatives

Some countries have implemented a safety radius for television and radio transmitters.

Below: *EMFs: A Factor in Road Rage? Power lines are often viewed as unsightly but seldom considered in relation to symptoms of anxiety, stress, and anger that we experience when we drive down the street.* **Credit**: *Angela Hobbs.*

Vehicles

The more whistles, buzzers, and bells a car has, the more it seems to appeal, from electric windows and doors, CD stackers, and loudspeakers in the headrest, to cruise control, electronic maps, and temperature sensors. The day when buying a car with an automatic transmission was the ultimate statement is long gone. Today our focus tends to be on gadgetry rather than on the safety of the environment in which we will spend hours cooped up. We spare little thought

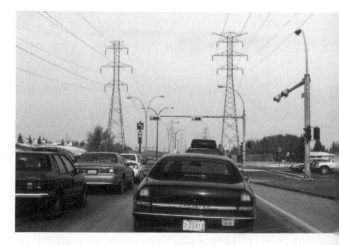

for the chemicals in the stain-resistant upholstery, rubberized car mats, carpets, and the foam in the seats. We think little of the EMFs from the LEDs that keep us informed of the temperature. We pay no attention to the EMFs produced by the brake disks in the wheels, or the wires that run through the seats to heat them, to deliver music to the head rest, or to preset the driving position for several different drivers.

When our bodies react to these environments with tingling feet, anxiety attacks, migraines, and road rage, we should examine the environment where they occur. Often the additional EMF load from roadside power lines, transmitters, and traffic lights compounds these symptoms. Society's unwillingness to recognize the possibility of an incompatibility with our immediate environment leaves some people refusing to go out, fearing the strange sensations that accompany every excursion.

Alternatives

If we want to be sure that the environment in which we will probably spend a couple of hours a day is compatible, we probably have to do without the whistles, buzzers, and bells. Roll-down windows may seem archaic to some, but they don't have EMFs. Not having a security system may seem like asking for trouble, but then maybe no one wants to steal a car with manual windows.

Computers

For some appliances there is no alternative: without them we cannot do our jobs. Of these, the computer is probably the most notable. When laptops were first introduced, people who had been alerted to the dangers of desktops breathed a sigh of relief. Unfortunately, the solution had not arrived. Many found their hands stiffening or tingling as they held them over the disk drives for hours at a time. Countless ergonomic chairs have been brought on to the market to quiet the concern over aching shoulders. It is still not generally accepted that our close proximity to the computer and monitor of the desktop, or to the hard drive and powerpack of the laptop computer, has any bearing upon the discomfort we feel. But keep in mind that the safety standards of the western world are based on the theory that

EMFs can do damage only if they cause heat at their point of impact, it should come as no surprise that we look everywhere for our solutions but at the electromagnetic fields around our computers. For many people who are sensitive to their computers, this general unwillingness to consider these EMF sources right under their noses leaves them thinking they must be going crazy. They're not!

Let's take a closer look at common symptoms experienced by people working on computer monitors, such as:

- pricking and burning sensations, often in the face and eyes;
- dry breathing passages;
- ear, nose, throat, and sinus problems that are not caused by viral or bacterial infections;
- difficulties with concentration, dizziness, and memory;
- headaches and nausea;
- teeth and jaw pains;
- aching muscles and joints;
- cardiac palpitations.

Fortunately there is something we can do to distance ourselves from the EMFs created by our computers.

Desktop

Increase the size of the desk so that the monitor can be pushed back, leaving the screen at least three feet from your face. Move the computer itself as far away as the wires will allow from where you are sitting when you use it. The EMFs from computers, like any electrical appliance, don't simply stop a couple of feet from the computer; pockets of EMF concentrations can be anywhere. If you are bothered by your symptoms after trying all the distancing suggestions, try changing the computer's location.

Laptop

The joy of the laptop is its convenience for use anytime, anywhere. The disk drive puts out significant EMFs — a feature we might want to take into consideration when we are going to use it for extended periods. To some, setting the laptop on a desk might seem to defeat its very purpose, but for others, setting the laptop on a desk and using an external keyboard and mouse creates a distance between the user and the disk drive's EMFs. The powerpack also creates EMFs. Often we plug the laptop into the most convenient outlet, leaving the powerpack to rest on our seat or at our feet. The use of an extension cord can change the location of the powerpack, again adding distance.

Airplanes can be very uncomfortable places if the person behind you is working on a laptop for hours at a time. Often the user will be willing to change places with you so that the laptop is not right up against your back. Television monitors and telephones in the headrest are becoming increasingly popular and until regulations catch up with this, the only alternative is to avoid airplanes that have them.

Shields

Efforts have been made to introduce some kind of shield to prevent EMFs from reaching our bodies. The chiropractor who first introduced me to electricity as a possible source of my problems suggested that sleeping on a specially-made lead plate would stop the EMFs from reaching my body. In actual fact, the range of EMFs that we're dealing with here is not as specific as those we are dealing with when we talk about X-rays — and though some might be blocked by lead, the vast majority would not.

The use of Mu-metal as an EMF shield has also been explored. Mu-metal is an alloy of nickel, iron, and some trace elements. Though Mu-metal is able to block EMFs, the frequency it blocks depends on the proportion of its ingredients and its thickness.

Mercury

Most checkups at the dentist include a panoramic X-ray, mouth X-rays, and bitewing X-rays to discover whether or not we need fillings. Once we discover that we do need fillings, we often want to get them done as quickly as we can. In the interests of business, dentists can be quite willing to "pop out the old, pop in the new, rinse and spit." Depending on the dentist, he may or may not be familiar with the dangers of mercury fillings or x-rays, and it may come as news to you that there is in fact a protocol for the removal of mercury amalgam fillings set by the International Academy of Oral Medicine and Toxicology (IAOMT). The vaporization of mercury that occurs when the drill, hot drinks, or simply chewing heats it causes the mercury levels in our mouths to exceed the air standards set by the US Environmental Protection Agency (EPA). The IAOMT's procedure protects everyone. The fillings

> Did you know that mercury is not only used in mercury amalgam fillings and encased in thermometers but also in the dyes used to color our hair and clothing, children's vaccinations,[7] and the glossy paper in magazines? The symptoms of mercury toxicity include headaches, nausea, arthritis, depression, muscle weakness, memory loss, etc.[8]

are kept cool with lots of cold water, the bits are suctioned with a high volume evacuator, large chinks are removed to minimize the surface area from which the mercury can vaporize, and an alternative air source limits how much vaporized mercury is breathed in.[6]

Of the mercury we absorb daily— from two to 15 micrograms — most comes from the amalgam fillings in our teeth. Contrary to popular belief, mercury is not stabilized by its combination with other metals.[9]

In Summary

Few people are in situations where moving is a viable option. We have to consider issues such as employment, the stake we have in our houses and communities, our proximity to family, etc. Most of us can't simply walk away. But if we find ourselves in a situation where we believe the overall level of EMFs from external uncontrollable sources such as power lines, cell phone base stations, and substations is at the root of our health problems or those of someone in our family, we may have no choice. The issues have to be weighed against the health of the person in our midst who is suffering. For their sake, we have to find a way to increase the amount of time they spend in an environment that gives their bodies a break. This may come in the form of changing from electric heating to either oil or gas. It may come in the form of having an electrician reroute the wires around and under their beds.

It may come in the form of moving their beds until we find a position in which they can fall asleep easily. It may come when we realize that the chair we ask them to sit in order to keep them ten feet from the television actually backs onto the dryer or stove, putting them within range of far greater EMFs than anything the television has to offer. It may come when we realize that our children are sitting in school all day next to old, substandard computers while we fret about the impact of the new power line.

Ultimately, the answers come to us as we view each source of EMFs and chemicals that place a burden on our bodies. We begin to see ways of eliminating them, and discover alternatives and strategies for distancing ourselves from the sources. The recognition that these seemingly innocuous sources are at the root of our problems is the first step in enabling us to deal with them one at a time. This change in perception is the biggest challenge of all.

Epilogue:
A New Beginning

To understand the man, we have to understand his world, the environment he lives in.
ARISTOTLE (C. 384–322 BC)

Y SEARCH FOR A SECOND OPINION initiated a journey of discovery and enlightenment. From being a mother who threw a cup of bleach into every wash and used tumble-dryer sheets with abandon, I became a mother who weighed the use of any chemical against its potential for harm.

There is no question that the road I traveled was arduous. The endless diagnoses and the testing required to confirm doctors' suspicions filled my days with fear and desperation, and the discomfort of the symptoms themselves left me exhausted and in pain. Often I prayed that my journey would be short: that I would find my second opinion and receive treatment. But had that been the case, I would never have learned what I did, and I probably wouldn't have been able to share my story with you.

From my first suspicions that my symptoms were somehow related to the smell in my house, the pressure mounted to convince me otherwise. Surrounded by friends and professionals who forcefully advocated their opinion that my symptoms were an expression of internal disease, I struggled to hold on to my wits. Despite the many differing diagnoses of the medical profession, the one thing they held in common was that my symptoms revealed that something was wrong with me. There was no support for the possibility that my symptoms might be a reaction to my environment.

With each diagnosis, I was introduced to another disease as the possible cause of my problems. My unwillingness to accept the diagnosis at face value led me to research it and in so doing I discovered much about real health that

I had never known. The most useful of all of these diagnoses was that of allergies. The treatment of allergies introduced me to the concept of eliminating things in my immediate environment that might be causing my symptoms. As I applied this knowledge to each factor in my environment, my path became clear. I ceased to be the victim and found confidence in myself as I discovered that I wasn't looking at just one burden in my environment but at all of them, at how they interacted with each other, and at how they interacted with me.

My path ultimately led me to realize that my symptoms were a product of my immediate environment. I gained an understanding of the way chemicals and EMFs affect the balance of my body and how I could regain this balance by controlling my exposure to them. Until I knew what I was doing wrong, I couldn't fix it. Once my body was balanced, the things that had once provoked symptoms no longer did. By taking control of my personal environment, I was able to create for myself a small world in which I was able to heal. From this controlled environment, I was able gradually to regain a normal life, one that includes all the things I was able to do before I got sick — working, traveling, parenting, swimming, hiking, camping, shopping, rollerblading, baking. The sky is again the limit.

Recognizing that I was incompatible with my environment was the key that unlocked the door to my recovery. There was never really anything wrong with me: my symptoms were warning signals. My body was telling me that I had created an environment that it was not created for. Removed from that environment and provided with an environment that it finds comfortable, my body no longer needs to send warning signals. It no longer needs to tell me to run!

Recommended Reading

Food – The Elimination Diet

William E. Walsh. *Food Allergies: The Complete Guide to Understanding and Relieving Your Food Allergies.* John Wiley & Sons, 2000.

In this book Dr. Walsh takes a detailed look at allergies to food chemicals. He leads us through avoidance, anticipated symptoms, the elimination diet, and even recipes. He discusses "additive" allergies and encourages readers to trust their instincts.

Theron G. Randolph and Ralph W. Moss. *An Alternative Approach to Allergies: The New Field of Clinical Ecology Unravels the Environmental Causes of Mental and Physical Ills.* Harper and Row Publishers, 1989.

Our susceptibility to the chemicals in our environment is the focus of this book, with the primary source being food. The Rotary Diversified Diet may help you track down foods responsible for your symptoms, and the comprehensive list of food groups in Appendix A may be useful if you're not sure which foods belong to which groups.

Gary Null. *No More Allergies: Identifying and Eliminating Allergies and Sensitivity Reactions to Everything in your Environment,* Random House, 1992.

Gary shows us how to use foods to build up our immune systems, offers a "no more allergies" diet and a selection of recipes. He tends to focus on foods as the culprit of reactions but also touches on ways we can clean up our environment.

Food – Additives

Russell L. Blaylock. *Excitotoxins: The Taste That Kills.* Health Press, 1996.

The author tells you all you need to know about excitotoxins — what they are, where to find them, and how they work.

EMFs

Mark A. Pinsky. *The EMF Book: What You Should Know About Electromagnetic Fields, Electromagnetic Radiation, and Your Health*. Warner Books, 1995.

Mark takes a look at the scientific research on electromagnetic fields, advising the reader which ones to be concerned about, and discusses the policies behind the siting of power lines and antennae in America.

Paul Brodeur approaches electromagnetic fields from the conspiracy angle in three books that are well worth reading if your curiosity about EMFs has been piqued, you're ready to be spooked, and are interested in knowing just how much effort our pioneers in the field of EMFs have had to put in to getting the word out.

The Zapping of America: Microwaves, Their Deadly Risk, and the Coverup. W.W. Norton and Company, 1977.

Currents of Death: Power Lines, Computer Terminals, and the Attempt to Cover Up Their Threat to Your Health. Simon and Schuster, 1989 (paperback 2001).

The Great Power-Line Cover-Up: How the Utilities and the Government Are Trying to Hide the Cancer Hazard Posed by Electromagnetic Fields. Little Brown & Company, 1993.

George Louis Carlos and Martin Schram. *Cell Phones: The Invisible Hazards of the Wireless Age: An Insider's Alarming Discoveries about Cancer and Genetic Damage*. Carroll and Graf, 2001.

The authors warn us as clearly as they can about the dangers of putting cell phones to our heads.

Nicholas H. Steneck. *The Microwave Debate*. The MIT Press, 1984.

The author offers a very balanced look at the early background of the debate regarding EMFs and health. Nicholas raises the question as to "whether the problems being addressed are amenable to narrow scientific solutions."

Alexander Pressman. *Electromagnetic Fields and Life*. Translated by F.L. Sinclair. Plenum, 1969.

This translation from the Russian will inform you about how much has been known about the effect of EMFs on physiology, and for how long. Pressman explained his theory before the world was ready to hear it.

Michael Milburn and Maren Oelbermann. *Electromagnetic Fields and Your Health: What You Need to Know About the Hidden Hazards of Electricity and How to Protect Yourself.* New Star Books, 1994.

This book gives an overview of the research into EMFs, the mechanisms by which EMFs impact our health, and some of the history behind the setting of exposure standards in the East and West.

Cyril W. Smith and Simon Best. *Electromagnetic Man: Health and Hazard in the Electrical Environment.* The Bath Press, 1989.

The authors take a look at the research that connects EMFs and ill-health.

EMFs and Hormones

T.S. Wiley. *Lights Out: Sleep, Sugar, and Survival.* Pocket Books, 2000.

This book reveals a great deal of insight into the impact on us of just one portion of the electromagnetic spectrum — light.

Russell J. Reiter and Jo Robinson. *Melatonin.* Bantam Books, 1996.

Just how important this hormone is to us, and not just in connection with cancer, is revealed by one of the world's leading experts.

Environment

Pavel Yutsis and Linda Toth. *Why Can't I Remember: Reversing Normal Memory Loss.* Avery, 1999.

This is an interesting read that takes us through memory disorders and the food additives and environmental pollutants that cause them. This book also looks at therapies that can lower toxicity levels — chelation and oxygen therapies, fasting, sauna, and Nambudripad's Allergy Elimination Technique (NAET) — and provides suggestions for steps we can take to improve memory.

John Harte, Cheryl Holden, Richard Schneider, and Christine Shirley. *Toxics A to Z: A Guide to Everyday Pollution Hazards.* University of California Press, 1991.

The authors spell out the sources, health and environmental effects, properties, regulatory status, and methods of prevention for a hundred or so common chemicals.

Environment – Building and Renovating

Paula Baker-Laporte, Erica Elliot, and John Banta. *Prescriptions for A Healthy House: A Practical Guide for Architects, Builders, and Homeowners*. New Society, 2001

The authors provide a low toxicity approach to renovating and building a house.

Maury Breechner and Shirley Linde, *Healthy Homes in a Toxic World: Preventing, Identifying, and Eliminating Health Hazards in Your Home*. John Wiley and Sons, 1992.

This book has a particularly useful list of helpful experts and agencies.

John Bower. *The Healthy House: How to Buy One, How to Build One, How to Cure a Sick One*. 4th edition. Healthy House Institute, 2000.

This book covers all aspects of the home, paying particular attention to lead, asbestos, radon, mold, combustion byproducts, and volatile organic compounds.

General Health

Andrew Weil. *Spontaneous Healing: How to Discover and Enhance Your Body's Natural Ability to Maintain and Heal Itself*. Ballantine Books, 1999.

This book illustrates the strength of our body's own healing mechanisms

Alternative Products

Debra Lynn Dadd. *Home Safe Home: Protecting Yourself and Your Family From Everyday Toxics and Harmful Products*. Jeremy P. Tarcher, 1997.

In her upbeat tone, Debra tells us what is bad for us, which alternatives work, where to get them, and how to make them.

Lynn Marie Bower. *The Healthy Household: A Complete Guide For Creating a Healthy Indoor Environment*. The Healthy House Institute, 1995.

This book's alternatives and methods tend to be geared towards people suffering from Multiple Chemical Sensitivities — everything from baking newspapers to portable saunas. Chapter 10 gives a comprehensive overview of the various forms of water treatment.

Annie Berthold-Bond. *Better Basics for the Home: Simple Solutions for Less Toxic Living*. Three Rivers Press, 1999.

This book offers many ideas to significantly reduce chemical exposure in the home.

Children's Health Environment Coalition. <www.Checnet.org>

Checnet has a "Virtual House" that allows you to click on the commodities to discover the dangers, the alternatives, and where to get them.

Multiple Chemical Sensitivity

Pamela Reed Gibson. *Multiple Chemical Sensitivities: A Survival Guide.* New Harbinger, 2000.

This book has interesting statistics on the various treatments used in dealing with MCS, revealing how many people they have helped and harmed. The first two parts give an overview of the characteristics, symptoms, causes, prevention methods, and treatments of MCS. Parts 3 and 4 reflect the prevailing attitude of the medical profession: MCS is a condition that we have to learn to live with, with little hope of recovery.

Endnotes

Introduction

1 United States General Accounting Office Report. *Indoor Pollution: Status of Federal Research Activities.* August 1999, p. 56

2 Ibid., p. 59

3 Polunin, Miriam, and Christopher Robbins. *The Natural Pharmacy: An Illustrated Guide to Natural Medicine.* Dorling Kindersley, 1992, p. 19

4 Blackwell, D.L. and J.F. Collins, R. Coles. "Summary Health Statistics for US Adults: National Health Interview Survey 1997." National Center for Health Statistics, Vital and Health Statistics Series 10, Data from National Health Survey Number 205, 2002, p. 4

Chapter 2

1 Environmental Protection Agency. [online] *Indoor Air Quality for Health Professionals.* 1989, p. 7 [Cited Apr. 10, 2002] <www.epa.gov/iaq/pubs/hpguide.html>

2 Harte, John, and Cheryl Holdren, Richard Sneider, Christine Shirley. *Toxics A to Z: A Guide to Everyday Pollution Hazards.* University of California Press, 1991, p. 318

3 Ibid., p. 326, p. 234, p. 215.

4 Putnam, Susan, and Jonathan Baert Weiner. [online] *Seeking Safe Drinking Water.* Harvard University Press, 1995, p. 4. [Cited Aug. 19, 2002] <http://c3.org/chlorine_knowledge_center/12749.html>

Chapter 3

1 Bullough, J., and M.S. Rea, R.G. Stevens. "Light and Magnetic Fields in a Neonatal Intensive Care Unit." *Bioelectromagnetics* Vol. 17(5), 1997, pp. 396–405

2 Sandström M, and E. Lyskov, A. Berglund, S. Medvedev, K. Mild. "Neurophysiological Effects of Flickering Light in Patients with Perceived Electrical Hypersensitivity." *Journal of Occupational and Environmental*

Medicine. Vol. 39, 1997, pp. 15–22. Cited in *NIEHS Report on Health Effects from Exposure to Power-Line Frequency Electric and Magnetic Fields.* Prepared in response to the 1992 Energy Policy Act. NIH Publication No. 99-4493, p. 19

3 United States General Accounting Office Report. *Indoor Pollution: Status of Federal Research Activities.* August 1999, p. 59

Chapter 5

1 Burch, J.D. and J.S. Reif, M.G. Yost, T.J. Keefe, C.A. Pittrat. "Nocturnal Excretion of a Urinary Melatonin Metabolite among Electric Utility Workers." *Scandinavian Journal of Work Environment Health.* Vol. 24(3), 1998, p.183–189

2 Carlo, George and Martin Schram. *Cell Phones: Invisible Hazards in the Wireless Age.* Carroll & Graf, 2001, p. 244

3 Balch, James F. and Phyllis A. Balch. *Prescription for Nutritional Healing.* Avery, 1997, p. 44, 57–58

4 Cherry, Neil. *Evidence that Electromagnetic Fields from High Voltage Power Lines and in Buildings Are Hazardous to Your Health, Especially to Very Young Children.* Environmental Management and Design Division, Lincoln University, New Zealand, 2001, p. 10

5 Wilson, B.W. and E.K Chess, L.E. Andersen. "60 Hz Electric Field Effects on Pineal Melatonin Rhythms." *Bioelectromagnetics* Vol. 7, 1986, p. 239–242. Cited in Jack M. Lee, Jr., *Electrical and Biological Effects of Transmission Lines; A Review.* Bonneville Power Adminsitration, 1996.

6 Södergren Leif. [online] *Hur Vår Miljö Kan Påverka Oss: Elöverkänslighet och Elva Pusselbitar. (How Our Environment Can Affect Us: Electrosensitivity and Eleven Puzzle Pieces).* FEB The Swedish Association for the Electrosensitive, 1998, p.9 [Cited Apr. 9, 1999] <www.feb.se/ARTICLES/MiljoeES.html>

7 Health Canada. [online] *The Health and Environment Handbook for Health Professionals.* Prepared by The Great Lakes United Health Effects Program, Ontario Ministry of Health, October 1997, Contaminant Profiles, Aluminum. [Cited Apr. 20, 2002] <www.hc.sc.gc.ca>

8 Ibid., Contaminant Profiles, Fluoride

9 Ibid., Contaminant Profiles, Fluoride

10 Ibid., p. 106

11 Ferrier, Catherine. [online] *Bottled Water: Understanding a Social Phenomenon. A discussion paper prepared for the World Wildlife Fund*, April 2001, p. 20 [Cited Apr. 4, 2002] <www.panda.org/livingwaters/pubs/bottled_water.pdf>

12 Health Canada. *The Health and Environment Handbook for Health Professionals.* p. 27

13 Kline, Monte. [online] *Shower Water Toxicity*. Pacific Health Center, Better Health Update No. 50, p. 3 [Cited Aug. 16, 2002] <www.pacifichealthcenter.com>

14 Yutsis, P., *Why Can't I Remember? Reversing Memory Loss*, p. 65

15 Ibid., p. 67

16 Sarasua, S. and D.A. Savitz. "Cured and Boiled Meat Consumption in Relation to Childhood Cancers." *U.S Cancer Causes and Control.* Vol.5, 1994, p. 141–148 Cited in Jack M. Lee, Jr., *Electrical and Biological Effects of Transmission Lines: A Review*. Bonneville Power Administration, 1996.

17 Health Canada. *The Health and Environment Handbook for Health Professionals.* Contaminant Profiles, Aluminum.

18 Morris, J. "Assessing Children's Toxic Risks: Pediatricians Gain New Diagnostic Tool." *U.S News and World Report*, October 18, 1999, p. 80

19 Lawson, Lynn. *Staying Well in a Toxic World: Understanding Environmental Illness, Multiple Chemical Sensitivities, Chemical Injuries and Sick Building Syndrome*. Noble Press, 1993, p. 250

20 Katzin, Carolyn. [online] *Fighting Cancer with a Fork*. The Cancer Nutrition Center, p. 1–2 [Cited Aug. 17, 2002] <www.cancernutrition.com/fork_lecture.htm>

21 Baer, Firman E. [online] *Variations in Mineral Content in Vegetables*. Rutgers University. Cited in Health and Freedom Resources Public Awareness Announcement No. 6, July 2000. [Cited Jul. 9, 2002] <www.healthfree.com/paa/paa0006.htm>

22 Health Canada. *The Health and Environment Handbook for Health Professionals*, October 1997, p. 143

23 Ibid., p. 144

24 Ebbert, Kristin. [online] "The Cosmetic Mask." *The Green Guide*, No. 31, November 1996, p. 3. [Cited Dec. 17, 2002] <www.thegreenguide.com>

25 Yutsis, P., *Why Can't I Remember? Reversing Memory Loss*, p. 73

26 Harte, J., *Toxics A to Z: A Guide to Everyday Pollution Hazards*, p. 308

27 Ibid., p. 435

28 Wallace, Lance. [online] *Identification of Polar Volatile Organic Compounds in Consumer Products and Common Microenvironments.* Environmental Protection Agency, 1991. Cited by Julia Kendall in *Fabric Softeners: Health Risks from Dryer Exhaust and Treated Fabrics.* [Cited Oct. 8, 2002] <www.herc.org/news/perfume/fabric.htm>

29 United States General Accounting Office Report. *Indoor Pollution: Status of Federal Research Activities.* August 1999, p. 4

30 Rousseau, David, and Jean Enwright, W.J. Rea. *Your Home, Your Health and Well-being.* Hartley and Marks, 1989. p. 43.

31 Södergren, L., *Hur Vår Miljö Kan Påverka Oss. Elöverkänslighet och Elva Pusselbitar. (How Our Environment Can Affect Us: Electrosentitivity and Eleven Puzzle Pieces),* p. 3

32 Renner, Rebecca. "Scotchgard Scotched: Following the Fabric Protectors Slippery Trail to A New Class of Pollutant." *Scientific American,* Vol. 284 (3), March 2001, p. 18

33 Harte, J., *Toxics A to Z: A Guide to Everyday Pollution Hazards,* p. 435

34 DeMatteo, Bob. *Terminal Shock.* New Canada Publications, 1985, p. 67–69

35 Steneck, Nicholas H. *The Microwave debate.* The Massachusetts Institute of Technology, 1984, p. 63

36 Becker, Robert O. *Cross Currents: The Perils of Electropollution, The Promise of Electromedicine.* Jeremy P. Tarcher, 1990, p. 248–266

37 O'Connor, Paul. *Multiple Sclerosis: The Facts You Need.* Canadian Medical Association, p. 14

Chapter 6

1 Morris, J., "Assessing Children's Toxic Risks: Pediatricians Gain New Diagnostic Tool" *US News and World Report,* October 18, 1999, p. 80

2 Ibid., p. 80

3 Yutsis, P., *Why Can't I Remember? Reversing Memory Loss,* p. 73

4 Reegan, Lisa. "What About Mercury? Getting Thimerosol Out of Vaccines." *Mothering,* March/April 2001, pp. 53–55

5 Murkerjee, M. "Superabsorbents." *Scientific American,* December 2000

6 Silny, J. *Effect of a 50 Hz Electric Field Influence on the Organism.* RGE-FRA. Special Issue 1976, pp. 81–90. Cited in the Review by Dr. Jack M. Lee, Jr., *Electrical and Biological Effects of Transmission Lines: A Review.* Bonneville Power Administration, 1996

7 Priesnitz, Wendy. Ed., [online] "Engineered Foods a Threat to Babies" *Natural Life Magazine* No. 68, p. 1 [Cited Aug. 16, 2002] <www.life.ca/na/68/babies.html>

8 Sharpe, Robert. *The Cruel Deception*. Thorsons (UK), 1988, p. 65

9 Lane, William I. and Linda Comac. *Sharks Still Don't Get Cancer*. Avery, 1996.

10 Glassner-Shwayder, Katherine. *Great Lakes Non-indigenous Invasive Species*. Briefing paper sponsored by the US Environmental Protection Agency, Office of Research and Development, and The Great Lakes National Program Office, 1999, p. 50

11 Ramirez, E., and J.Z. Monteagudo, G. Garcia, J.M.R. Delgado, "On Position and Development of Drosophila Modified by Magnetic Fields." *Bioelectromagnetics* 4, p. 315–326

12 Ryle, Sarah. [online] *Insurers Balk at Risks of Phones*. From *The Observer*, London, UK, April 11, 1999. [Cited in Wave Guide.org] <www.wave-guide.org/news/lloyds.html>

Chapter 7

1 Young, Louise B. *Power Over People*. Oxford University Press, 1992, p. 19

2 Bonneville Power Administration. *Electrical and Biological Effects of Transmission Lines: A Review*. Prepared by Dr. Jack M. Lee, Jr., 1996, p. 1–2

3 *WHO Information Fact Sheet*, No. 193, June 2000

4 Santini, R. and M. Seigne, L. Bonhomme-Faivre. "Danger of Cell Phones and Their Relay Stations." *Pathol Biol*. Vol. 48 (6) 2000, p. 525–528

5 The Swedish Association for the Electrosensitive. [online] *Switzerland Adopts Strict Limits for Cell Towers and Power Lines*. News Archive 1999–2000, Feb. 1, 2000 [Cited Aug. 16, 2001] <www.feb.se/NEWS/index.html>

6 International Academy of Oral Medicine and Toxicology. [online] *Protocol for Mercury and Silver Filling Removal*. [Cited Sept. 13, 1999] <http://emporium.turnpike.net/p/pdha/mercury/iaomt.htm>

7 Morris, J., *Assessing Children's Toxic Risks*, p. 80

8 Harte, J., *Toxics A to Z: A Guide to Everyday Pollution Hazards*, p. 342

9 Yutsis, P., *Why Can't I Remember? Reversing Memory Loss*, pp. 65–67

Index

About the Author

Angela Hobbs *(née von Sicard)* was raised in Arusha, Tanzania, Uppsala in Sweden, and Birmingham, England. After studying in Strasbourg, France, and Link^ping, Sweden, Angela graduated from the Universities of East Anglia and Central England. Her teaching career, and a keen interest in cultural diversity, took Angela from the language schools of Frankfurt, Germany to England's village schools and Arctic Quebec. When a sick house brought her life to a standstill, Angela immersed herself in five years of researching the sick house and chemical and electromagnetic sensitivities. Today, fully recovered, Angela works as a researcher and as a substitute teacher specializing in Learning Disabilities, Music and English as a Second Language. She lives with her husband and two children in Calgary, Alberta.

Prescriptions for A Healthy House

A Practical Guide for Architects, Builders, & Homeowners

Paula Baker-Laporte, Erica Elliott and John Banta

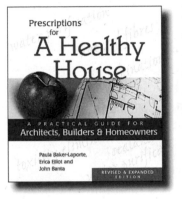

For people concerned about exposure to toxins found in conventional building materials and practices, this invaluable guide explains why standard building practices are not healthful, shows how to design interior and exterior space and select construction materials that promote physical well-being, and how to obtain alternative materials and expertise.

336 PAGES 8 X 9"

50 B&W ILLUSTRATIONS AND PHOTOGRAPHS

ISBN 0-86571-434-7

US$26.95 / CAN$36.95

The Art of Natural Building

Design, Construction, Resources

Joseph E. Kennedy, Michael G. Smith and Catherine Wanek, Editors

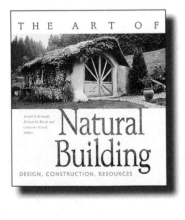

An encyclopedia of natural building for non-professionals as well as architects and designers, this anthology of articles from leaders in the field covers straw bale and cob, through recycled concrete and salvaged materials, focusing on both the practical and the esthetic concerns of ecological building designs and techniques.

288 PAGES 8 X 9"

200 B&W PHOTOGRAPHS & DRAWINGS

8 PAGE FULL-COLOR SECTION

ISBN 0-86571-433-9

US$26.95 / CAN$36.95

The Natural Plaster Book

Earth, Lime and Gypsum Plasters for Natural Homes

Cedar Rose Guelberth and Dan Chiras

This unique step-by-step guide takes the confusion out of choosing, mixing, and applying natural plasters and is written for the growing number of people who have decided to build their own natural homes (of straw bale, cob, adobe, rammed earth, and other natural materials), as well as for professionals. Heavily illustrated with practical drawings and photographs, it also includes an extensive resource guide listing books, magazines, videos, builders, and suppliers.

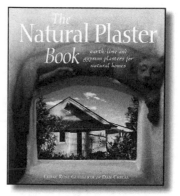

304 PAGES 8 x 9"

ISBN 0-86571-449-5

US$29.95 / CAN$44.95

Straw Bale Building

How to Plan, Design, and Build with Straw

Chris Magwood and Peter Mack

Straw Bale Building leads the potential builder through the entire process of building a bale structure, tackling all the practical issues from how to find and choose bales; developing sound building plans; costs; roofing; electrical, plumbing, and heating systems; building code compliance and working with building inspectors; and special concerns for builders in northern climates.

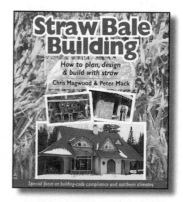

256 PAGES 8‰ x 9‰

ARCHITECTURAL DRAWINGS & B&W PHOTOS

ISBN 0-86571-403-7

US$24.95 / CAN$29.95

If you have enjoyed *The Sick House Survival Guide* you might also enjoy other

BOOKS TO BUILD A NEW SOCIETY

Our books provide positive solutions for people who want to make a difference. We specialize in:

Sustainable Living • Ecological Design and Planning • Natural Building & Appropriate Technology
New Forestry • Environment and Justice • Conscientious Commerce • Progressive Leadership
Educational and Parenting Resources • Resistance and Community • Nonviolence

For a full list of NSP's titles, please call 1-800-567-6772 or check out our web site at:
www.newsociety.com

New Society Publishers

ENVIRONMENTAL BENEFITS STATEMENT

New Society Publishers has chosen to produce this book on New Leaf EcoBook 100, recycled paper made with 100% post consumer waste, processed chlorine free, and old growth free.

For every 5,000 books printed, New Society saves the following resources:[1]

33	Trees
3,011	Pounds of Solid Waste
3,313	Gallons of Water
4,321	Kilowatt Hours of Electricity
5,474	Pounds of Greenhouse Gases
24	Pounds of HAPs, VOCs, and AOX Combined
8	Cubic Yards of Landfill Space

---

[1]Environmental benefits are calculated based on research done by the Environmental Defense Fund and other members of the Paper Task Force who study the environmental impacts of the paper industry.

For more information on this environmental benefits statement, or to inquire about environmentally friendly papers, please contact New Leaf Paper – info@newleafpaper.com Tel: 888 • 989 • 5323.

NEW SOCIETY PUBLISHERS